Amorous Initiation

AMOROUS

INITIATION

A Novel of Sacred and Profane Love

An excerpt from the Memoirs
of the Chevalier Waldemar de L———

O. V. de L. Milosz

Translated by Belle N. Burke

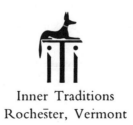

Inner Traditions
Rochester, Vermont

Inner Traditions International
One Park Street
Rochester, Vermont 05767

First published in English in 1994 by Inner Traditions

First published in French under the title *L'Amoureuse Initiation* by
Bernard Grasset, Paris, 1910

Copyright © 1958 by Editions André Silvaire

Translation copyright © 1994 by Inner Traditions International

Library of Congress Cataloging-in-Publication Data
Milosz, O. V. de L. (Oscar Vladislas de Lubicz), 1877–1939.
[Amoureuse initiation. English]
The amorous initiation : a novel of sacred and profane love /
O. V. de L. Milosz. — 1st English ed.
p.   cm.
ISBN 0-89281-418-7
I. Title.
PQ2625.I558A6513   1994
843'.912—dc20   93-30584
                                                                            CIP

Printed and bound in the United States

10 9 8 7 6 5 4 3 2 1

Text design by Charlotte Tyler

Distributed to the book trade in the United States
by American International Distribution Corporation (AIDC)

Distributed to the book trade in Canada
by Publishers Group West (PGW), Montreal West, Quebec

Distributed to the book trade in the United Kingdom
by Deep Books, London

Distributed to the book trade in Australia
by Millennium Books, Newtown, N. S. W.

Illustration on page 2: Interior of St. Marks, Venice. Etching by Otto-Henry
Bacher (1856–1909). Reproduced courtesy of The Metropolitan Museum of Art.
Gift of Mrs. Otto H. Bacher, 1932.

Foreword

Many years ago in Paris I met my relative, the author of this novel. I was a young student then, and that meeting proved to be the beginning of a lifelong fascination with his personality and his *oeuvre*. His influence has since been always present in my own literary work. This foreword is one of the tokens of my lasting gratitude. He taught me respect for all beings and things of this earth and at the same time tried to help me assess critically the modes of thought and belief of our century. That was a salutary preparation of my young mind for the time of horror and confusion in Europe, and I was to discover that in many hopeless situations the memory of his writings and of our conversations was able to protect me from despair.

A strange origin and a strange life. Deeply attached to France and masterful in the handling of various styles in French, Oskar

Wladyslaw Milosz was not a born Frenchman. He was born in 1877 on his hereditary estate in the former Grand Duchy of Lithuania, today the territory of Lithuania and Belarus. Brought up in Paris, cosmopolitan, traveling in many countries, and speaking several languages, he became a French poet under the name of Oscar V. de L. Milosz and an explorer of mystical realms little known to his contemporaries. *Amorous Initiation,* published in 1910, has justly been hailed as one of the great love stories of French literature, yet for its author it marked a stage in his incessant search for "the Love that moves the sun and the other stars." The novel brings to our mind Dante, though in it a Venetian courtesan takes the place of Beatrice. The realization of the unity of the sensual and the spiritual, as in the biblical Song of Songs, leads the narrator to a higher state of consciousness and to contemplation of the Divine discernible in Creation.

His 1912 mystery play, *Miguel Mañara,* tells about the ascent of a Spanish libertine and debauchee to sainthood through his love for a woman after he loses her to death. That work was followed by a most fruitful period in Milosz's poetry. Written mostly in "versets" (i.e., biblical verses), these poems describe the desolate landscapes of big cities and are like the prayers of a solitary man. This period in his life was a preparatory stage for an extraordinary experience of mystical initiation in December 1914, so powerful that he would soon abandon poetry and dedicate himself to presenting his prophetic vision in two treatises, or rather metaphysical poems, *Ars Magna,* 1924, and *Les Arcanes (The Arcana),* 1927.

An American reader interested in this extraordinary man and his works will find translations of his poems (some done as early as 1914) by Ezra Pound, Kenneth Rexroth, David Gascoyne, Christopher Bamford, Eduard Roditi, and John Peck. A substantial volume of Milosz's writings, both poems and treatises, entitled *The Noble Traveller,* edited and selected by Christopher Bamford with my introduction, appeared in 1985 (Inner Traditions/Lindisfarne Press). Philip Sherrard attempts to explain the importance of Milosz's approach to science in his book *Human Image: World Image. The Death and Resurrection of Sacred Cosmology* (Ipswich, U.K.: Golgonooza Press, 1992).

It would not be correct to see in Milosz a literary figure only, just as it would be wrong to treat William Blake in that manner. Certain affinities of his thought with that of Blake are intriguing, especially since he was not familiar with the English poet. Blake rejected Newtonian physics as evil and fumed at the "diabolical" triad of Bacon, Locke, and Newton. Similarly, Milosz held the "false physics" of Newton responsible for the sterile image of the cosmos exerting its destructive power on the human soul and making humanity homeless in the universe. Unlike Blake, he found an ally in contemporary physics. He considered Einstein's concept of space and time to be not only a revolution in science but also a discovery in the religious sense, leading to a new era, to a spiritual Renaissance. Milosz predicted that humanity would move toward a completely new science and, helped by it, would recover the harmony between religion, science, and art. Commentator Philip Sherrard writes, "The idea of space—the idea of space extended to infinity—and its corresponding idea of an eternity of succession divided into past, present, and future are indeed, as Milosz states, Satan himself in all the immense black majesty of its terrors."

Deliberately following in the steps of alchemists, Milosz revindicates some ideas of Paracelsus and of Jakob Boehme as well as those of the Kabbalah, seeing throughout human history a hidden thread of sacred knowledge. Yet his metaphysical treatises of poems are, above all, hymns praising the all-pervading power of love and the divine sacrifice through the Incarnation. Thus his philosophy is but a development of what we already find in his novel.

He was an attentive reader of Swedenborg but not quite in agreement with him; here is one more analogy with William Blake. From Swedenborg he borrowed the use of a Greek word, *Storge,* which means the love of parents for their children. Under Milosz's pen, Storge was his love for humans; he called it "an ancient love worn down by pity, anger, and solitude." He tried to serve his fellow men as well as he could and after World War I chose diplomacy as his field of activity. As his father's family had come from the area of ethnic Lithuania (his mother was Jewish and from Warsaw), he called himself a Lithuanian poet of the French language and served the newly independent country of his paternal ancestors as a member of the Lithuanian delegation to the League of Nations and as the first representative of Lithuania in Paris. His tomb—in Fontainebleau, where he died in the spring of 1939—bears an inscription in two languages, French and Lithuanian.

Czeslaw Milosz
Berkeley, California
August 1993

AMOROUS INITIATION

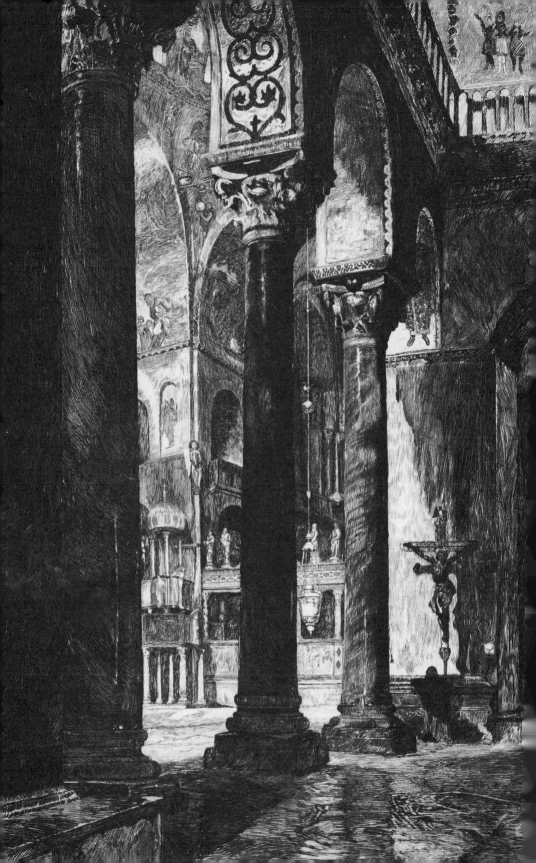

I N READING THIS
faithful account of my adventures, one may notice more than
once how little it costs me, at the end of my life, to acknowledge the mediocrity of the role I have played in this world. It
would be unjust, however, to attribute to pettiness of heart or
mind that which I believe is only the very natural result of experience and disenchantment. There was a time when I thought
of nothing else but to prepare myself for the noble career to
which my birth and my natural talents appeared to call me; a
time when I used to abandon myself only too willingly to dreams
of glory and dedication that, later on, grudging reality taught
me so well were of little importance; a time . . . a time far away,
lost, forever flown!

One day I awoke, bemused, to the realization of my true
destiny, and recognized myself to be one of those unfortunate

souls in whom the burning imagination of adolescence consumes the reality of an entire life. Nevertheless, shaking off my lethargy, I resigned myself as best I could, made my entrance on stage—and the show began. A pitiful tragicomedy! What can I tell you about it that you do not already know? I have never been able to play anything more than a supporting character in it, one of the most inconspicuous, and no doubt I shall die without ever having known its hero. Nothing is more difficult than learning to play the leading role in the events of one's own life. Have I loved, have I hated? I remember having laughed and cried; but never have I felt beneath my hand the beating of the heart, whether lacerated or joyful, of reality. In a way, I have lived only in order to have something to survive. As I write these futile recollections, I am aware of accomplishing the most important act of my life. I was predestined for Memory.

As mediocre as my opinion of my character may be, it becomes a kind of panegyric compared to the little confidence I place in my merits as a writer. If it is sometimes good to unite two personalities in oneself, it is always hateful to have a different style for each; but what could resemble the expression of my thought less than the language of my emotions? I find in all my writings the same disturbing mark of a collaboration between warring brothers. In addition, I share the great defect common to most sons of the North, that of respecting truth too much and neglecting grace. Should one merely touch on a subject or approach it with caution? Immediately I fly straight at it, like a starling to birdlime. Is it a question, on the other hand, of illustrating a noble or pleasant feature? Then I stop, hesitate for a long time, and retreat in great embarrassment, much like a timorous bear cub in front of a hive sparkling with honey and empty of bees. Finally, I am more content to evoke fortuitous happenings than to recall the few rare triumphs of my will or of my intelligence, and I consider myself so lacking in a sense of order and continuity that the moment I have reason to feel dissatisfied with the arrangement of one part I abandon everything to chance, the result being the confusion and dislocation for which I am so often and so rightly blamed.

Allow me, however, to note in my defense how difficult it is to arrange in order events whose relationship one tries in vain to discover. I cannot remember one occasion where I have not been the plaything of fate. The unforeseen has ruled my life like a tyrant who is both cruel and facetious, and I do not believe I have ever followed any rule of conduct other than to submit sadly to its capricious decrees.

Besides, dear reader, you have known for a long time now the persecutor of the unfortunate Benjamin. The strange eccentricity of his moods can no longer surprise you, any more than the sometimes inapt grotesquery of the disguises he was in the habit of assuming. I might have even more than one reason to suspect you of a secret indulgence toward this sly Chance, the enemy of my tranquility; yet I cannot avoid a feeling of uneasiness at the memory of the repulsive face it pleased him to wear for an encounter in Naples, toward the end of the year 17—after my return from Formosa. I will never obliterate from my memory the ludicrous details of that adventure. Despite the long lapse of time dividing me from it and the friendship which I have felt since then for its strange hero, I blush to confess that I owe the acquaintance of the most agreeable of the odd characters met in the course of my wandering life to the fury of a starving, mangy cur. It is only right, however, that in this instance the sentiment of gratitude take precedence over a vain preoccupation with the proprieties; for if the belligerence of the dreadful animal had not caused me to stumble on a cutthroat's doorstep, I should never have seen the ghostly silhouette of Count Pinamonte stop, in the middle of the night and of the Ponte Tappio, or turn toward me, in the winking light of a gambling house, the startling face of the last of the Benedettos.

At the end of this combat without honor, I was looking for my hat on the wet pavement of the dark alley where it had rolled, when suddenly I noticed an extraordinary, agitated figure at once arrogant and timid. Despite the hour and the place, the stranger was courteous enough to pick up my hat and to take off his own in greeting, so that his hands were holding two hats at once. We looked at each other in silence for a while. That first impression remains etched deep in my mind, for it gave birth to a very peculiar idea which torments me still today: certain encounters never happen for the first time, and there are in this world people and objects one would swear to having known for all eternity. I regarded the stranger with surprise and not without some distrust; for his part, he looked my tottering person up and down with a gaze steeped in astonishment and malice. . . .

"Well, by the great Devil!" he exclaimed at last. "Hang all hypocritical reserve! Beneath the disarray of your clothes I divine a man of superior quality; even your wine, if you don't mind my saying so, has the odor of good company. I am bored to death tonight, my dear sir; therefore, welcome!"

His voice—the grating, rusty voice of a March weathervane—seemed to me to be full of forced gaiety, poorly disguised faintheartedness, and a kind of sickly sanctimoniousness that gave it uncertain and shifting inflections. I took my hat from the emaciated, trembling hands of this remarkable individual and stammered, by way of thanks and introduction, my title, accompanied by the name of one of my domains.

"Well, by the Styx! look what's emerged from a Danish coat of arms! From what I see of you . . . no! I don't believe I've had the honor of meeting you; just the same, your face is not unknown to me. Which is not to say, chevalier, that I recall having seen it, but those eyes remind me of many, even of too many, things . . . I am Sassolo Sinibaldo, Count Pinamonte and thirteenth Duke of Brettinoro. My friend Poniatowski,* the philosopher king, calls me, for reasons I should find it difficult to explain, Count-Duke Antisthène.* My grandmother was a Guidoguerra, and sometimes, when I've drunk too much, I catch myself being proud of the ties that bind me to the extinct house of Benedetto."

The howls of my starving, mangy cur could still be heard, fading away; at intervals, a raucous tomcat added his amorous lament to the mournful tones of that gaming-house Cerberus. A pungent liquid fell from a window onto the slimy pavement. A clock struck, the hour uncertain in the suddenly deeper gloom foreshadowing the dawn. I scrutinized my talkative acquaintance. As emaciated and stooped as he was, he appeared to be fairly well built; but his face, which age had carved into great folds and on which the memory of his worst day seemed to have hardened into a bittersweet grimace both tearful and mirthful, made me shiver with pity and disgust. Drawn wrinkles ran in all directions on a bloodless face marked by random evil; curious twitchings of a large nose swollen with circumspect arrogance divulged the habit, common to nomads, of sniffing the air of various countries; the eyes vile and inquisitive (in Sumatra I saw a race of gigantic frugivorous rats whose glance, blazing with hideous wisdom, made my gorge rise), the restless, shifting eyes of my new friend froze from time to time in a kind of burning, empty fixity which congealed my blood.

M. de Pinamonte continued to babble. I would not even attempt to describe the frantic flight of his speech or the violence of his gesturing. Although there was very little continuity in all this verbiage, to which I paid only partial attention, I couldn't help experiencing a certain pleasure, combined with anguish, as I listened. For, apart from their meaning, words and inflections caressed my soul in the same manner as the strains of an old song heard long ago in the world of childhood. I was extraordinarily interested in my strange companion, recognizing him to be one of those somewhat mad coxcombs who see themselves less in mirrors than in the idea which they have of themselves; a secretive, fanciful breed, yet reliable, for their pride is the chief guarantee of their sincerity. This one, I thought, is too fond of himself not to appear as the world has made him. If he lies, it is only to flirt with himself, for he doubtless considers any truth good enough for his hearers. I noticed too that his extremely high birth was much more a subject of poetic reverie for him than an actual situation with which to feed his vanity. His singular wit made me think of a serpent's fascinating and repellent grace, but taken as a whole he reminded me most of all of the large ravens of my country which are at the

8

same time hideous and beautiful, comical and sinister. Two little furrows of tenderness played at the corners of the wide mouth that was almost too flexible and mobile, softening somewhat the harshness of his long, ravaged face from which all light had fled.

The moral nature of my great devil of an Antisthène appeared to me to be that of a lucid and argumentative sentimentalist, iniquitous because of his disgust for the world rather than by nature. His casual attire, slightly dusty and rumpled, was in remarkable harmony with the singularly attractive ugliness of his face, as well as with the alternately indolent and sudden movements of his tall, ungainly body—perhaps because I guessed the contemptuous negligence of his outfit to be deliberate without sacrificing anything of its naturalness. The creases of an article of clothing are sometimes the prolongation of certain facial lines, and those which I observed in the Neapolitan's clothes struck me as the expression of moral disillusionment much more than of physical indifference.

M. de Pinamonte was dressed in the manner of those who live too long in seclusion with their souls. I inspected my odd friend's loose-fitting black trousers, his unpowdered peruke, the jacket cut in the style of the past century, and his deplorable jabot, and my impression was that I had suddenly awakened in an unknown world ruled only by feelings, hostile to gloomy, sterile human reason. All the components of this bizarre personage—the magnetic stare of a nocturnal rodent, his voice, rusty as an old weathercock, the crackled parchment of his long, sharp face, his simpering, facetious melancholy, finally, his walk, which changed abruptly from a solemn pace to a trot, and everything else as well, including that insolent way of tapping his cheek with a moist, wrinkled suede glove that resembled a dead bat—yes, all the details of this extraordinary figure dissolved into a kind of fantastic harmony, an incoherent totality that revealed a remarkable unity of temperament beneath the diverse manifestations of ideas and moods.

My eyes hardly left the inexhaustible chatterer, yet, in spite of the bright light already shining on everything around us, it seemed as if the count-duke preferred to evade my scrutiny. To my inner eye he was enigmatic and vague; as I perceived him through the thin but deep mist of dreams and feelings which his presence aroused in the very pit of my being, he was like a silent spider seen through the gossamer of its web, or like the inhabitants of an aquarium, nourishing themselves on stillness in the cloud of their own externalized mystery. Far from revealing his soul, his flow of words seemed to conceal his thoughts. He intoxicated himself with idle chatter as other wretches become drunk on liquor. All his being breathed haste, uneasiness; his walk was as lively as his speech, and I had trouble keeping up with him. A mute automaton, I practically ran after him through the deserted streets. I had nothing to ask and nothing to answer; I was like a man who has just awakened from sleep and awaits the clarification of a great mystery.

A little beggar squatting on the steps of a church implored us with her consumptive eyes and held out her wooden bowl for alms. Antisthène halted his fitful gait at once, pulled out a miser's frayed purse, and, slipping a gold coin into the empty bowl, spoke into the child's ear a few words that struck me as a suspicious proposition. A hiccough of wine and disgust escaped from my lips. The uneasy, empty sun of insomnia shivered miserably on the muddy pavement.

Outraged by the manners of my peculiar acquaintance, I indicated my wish to part company and raised my hand to my hat. But Pinamonte, shaking with sudden laughter and holding my arm, exclaimed, "That was to test you! On my honor, chevalier, what a curious man you are! I should have believed you to be more disabused in worldly matters; who could you be but someone who has survived for the sake of revenge? Tell me the truth: for believe me, parricide, incest, rape, arson, and poisoning are implicit in the most ingenuous or the most inoffensive lie."

Then, this fantastic person punctuated his diabolical peroration by making a loud, wet noise with his tongue and let it be understood, with an obvious and comical wink of his eye and of his entire face, that only he, Sassolo Sinibaldo, Count Pinamonte and thirteenth Duke of Brettinoro, had arrived at this lamentable knowledge of man's heart and mind. I stared with surprise and not without a kind of startled sympathy at the garrulous old man, who was now occupied in lifting toward the morning sky the severe, facetious index finger of an apostle; I suddenly began to laugh with a childlike freshness that astonished my own ears. Far from being offended by this sudden attack of merriment, Antisthène echoed it in the freest and most gracious manner possible, with the result that we continued happily on our way, arm in arm. "Would you deign to honor my modest abode with your presence?" Doubtless noticing a glimmer of indecision in my eyes, he then said, "Set your mind at ease, chevalier. I live in the family home of the Brettinoros, which is in a quiet, secluded section; the old house is filled with restful, modest, discreet objects among which there is little chance, I believe, of your not feeling at home. We'll have some coffee and chat about whatever interests you; among the thousand charming objects with which my home is furnished you're sure to find something to your taste. I feel drawn to you by a feeling which is still obscure, but whose motive we cannot fail to discover sooner or later. Something about you speaks to me of the most precious moments of my past life. By Cain in the moon spots! Where have I seen them before, those eyes which seem never to have contemplated life's horrible nakedness? I have so many things to tell you! Ah, sweet sorceress, concubine of the Devil! So many years lost, so many illusions slaughtered! O my love! O most poisonous of hell's reptiles! . . . Look!" he exclaimed abruptly, pointing to a noble old house half covered by thick autumn foliage. "Chance has led you to my home. For the pleasant ruin before you bears the pompous name of Palazzo Brettinoro. Just one moment, no more, and I shall be completely at your service, body and soul, chevalier!"

While still talking, my Antisthène imperceptibly had moved some steps away, and now I watched him as, lifting high in the manner of a dog a leg thin as that of an old dancing master, he hastily watered the leprous wall of his garden. I looked up. The windows of the Brettinoro mansion reminded me of the veiled appearance of eyes suffering from a mortal affliction. In the precise center of the main door a scamp had traced in chalk the insolent curve of a Titan's natural attributes. My glance wandered distractedly over the somber facade, the sight of which was chilling. Sighing, I murmured the name of my dead lady of Vercelli. At that hour all was cool and rustling, yet everything appeared to me to be drowned in the mist of an endless melancholy that, following my shadow wherever it went, had long since overwhelmed me with a feeling of extreme age and of unbearable desolation. A sickly Jew's-harp mewed somewhere in the distance, the romantic song of an Italy gone forever. It was the voice of the past, of oblivion, and of solitude, to be sure; but still it was a voice, and my plaintive friend of Vercelli had been for ten years the inhabitant of a distant region inhospitable to any echo.

It was not without a certain emotion that I felt the first whiff of mephitic air catch in my throat in the dilapidated entrance hall of Palazzo Brettinoro. The mossy, somnolent odor of old homes is the same in all countries, and in the course of my solitary pilgrimages to the holy places of memory and nostalgia, closing my eyes in some antiquated house was enough to take me back instantly to the gloomy residence of my Danish ancestors, and to relive in the space of a moment all of the joys and sorrows of a childhood accustomed to the gentle aroma, so full of rain and twilight, of ancient abodes.

Forgetting the presence of the ironic Antisthène, once more I let myself surrender to the temptation of summoning the mysterious charm of bygone days; closing my eyes, I inhaled lovingly the stagnant mustiness of the palace. This act had always seemed to me completely natural, yet it provoked my host to excessive hilarity; this devil of an Antisthène immediately began to laugh, sneeze, cough, and spit all at once, to the great indignation of a trio of shabby, decrepit knaves who appeared without warning, dressed in hospital shirts and threadbare livery breeches.

"Before you review, according to ancient custom, all of the family portraits that inhabit this horrible place, chevalier, permit me to present the shameless rascals whom you see before you, for certainly they are more familiar to me than the foolish or abject faces that decorate the walls of my home. Here you have Giovanni, Francesco, and Pietro, servants equal to the best exemplars of the last century. Although they brought my fop of a father all the gossip of the streets and shops, they were very careful not to mention in his presence certain nocturnal frolics in which the ladies of our house played opposite them; therefore, they seem to me well deserving of the attentions and honors the offspring of their former masters bestows on them in their old age."

As impassive as they were deplorable, the servants condescended to answer the satiric jests of the old man only by bowing deeply with stern grace, after which they ceremoniously retired, walking backward. This beautiful gravity, so full of mute reproach, did not fail to produce the effect I expected: an abrupt reversal of my host's mood. Already I had every reason in the world to think that the whimsical exuberance of the count-duke was anything but his natural disposition; at first sight, I had guessed this unique person to be an unhappy and timorous soul. Accordingly, as soon as the door had closed behind the servants, M. de Pinamonte showed the degree of his agitation. Lowering his eyes, furiously rubbing his temples, coughing, sighing, and grumbling all together, he led me into the portrait gallery of his ancestors, where the one who had the misfortune to first greet our view immediately received, in a direct hit on his armor, all the ammunition of trinkets, keys, coins, and snuff boxes that distended the pockets of his irascible and fearful descendant. No doubt completely astonished by the great military feat he had just accomplished, and suddenly at peace again, the last of the Brettinoros pirouetted elegantly and in the calmest way possible began to tell me the history of the ancestor whose dumbfounded martial face he had just abused.

I only half-listened to the eloquence of my chance friend, my attention having been caught by a painting relegated to the darkest corner of the gallery. It was the portrait of a young woman, whose sorrowful look quickly aroused the cruelest memories in my heart.

"And the one you see here," continued the sadistic Antisthène, ". . . but what the deuce are you looking at, chevalier? Here, look, this long, livid, penitent's face, this cardinalized Satan, is Lotto Pinamonte the Treacherous, who made his father, Lorenzo, eat the fruits of Brother Albéric.* The beautiful lady whom you see over there was Adelasia Brettinoro, the passionate one whose jealous tongue never wearied of replenishing Abélard's brotherhood; and here is Ezzolino de Guidoguerra, called the Libicocco, the same man who, one beautiful summer evening, deemed it gallant to consume the heart of his own daughter, Gentucca, in an incestuous frenzy."

To no avail I pretended to be attentive or simulated interest or credulity; the indifference of the glances which, purely from courtesy, I cast from time to time at the malefactors of the house of Brettinoro did not escape the vigilance of their shrewd descendant.

Laughing, he said, "Nothing is so easily discovered as the reason for unmotivated sadness. However, do not let it disturb you, my friend, for I have not the slightest wish to scoff at a distraction that proves so well the sureness of your taste. The portrait that fascinates you bears the extremely rare signature of Sassolo Sinibaldo Pinamonte; as for the young lady whose beauty he gives himself the honor to present to you, know that she was a powerful and perfidious magician whose story, sad as well as salacious, will certainly figure in your entertainment presently. Meanwhile," he went on, striking his forehead as if inspired, "an excellent idea has come to me, a luminous idea; I might even say divine. Yes, by the Devil, divine! Giovanni will set up a small table right now in this very gallery and, while we restore the energies depleted by last night's amorous or bacchanalian adventures, we will evoke, in front of the portrait of the bewitching Manto, the charm of dead illusions and buried hopes. By the Brettinoros! It will be mournful, sportive, and delightful. I run, I fly to give the necessary orders."

The indefatigable talker, setting in motion the impatient springs of his long, elegant legs, disappeared as if by magic in the eddies of an antique tapestry whose sudden movement blinded me with a dusty shower of mummified gadflies and spiders' webs.

I could not even begin to describe the disquiet that overwhelmed me in the instant when, approaching the sorceress, I thought that I recognized in her face the large and ardent eyes of her who had been my soul and who for the past ten years had been sleeping beneath the distant cypresses of Vercelli. I leave it to the reader to imagine my painful surprise; no doubt it will be very easy for him if he is at all sensitive, for the sighs that escaped me resembled in every particular those which he himself would have breathed during a similar experience. After the first shock I regained some control over my emotions and, looking away from the disturbing eyes of the enchantress, studied her entire person.

As this obliged me to realize that she was completely foreign to me, I was not slow to feel some disenchantment with certain of her disproportions. The impudent line of her chin was not at all in harmony with the almost supernatural slenderness of the unknown woman; the oddly joined lines of the long, receding ears gave her face a bizarre, indescribable expression, uneasy and wild as a wary animal crouching in shadow; and it seemed to me that I saw in the cruel, unhappy curve of her lower lip, as well as in the low, shadowed brow, a confession of the most dreadful instincts and the mark of the direst recollections.

Completely rid of my preoccupation, I pulled open the dusty curtain that filtered the light from one of the gallery's high windows and could not suppress an exclamation of surprise on seeing by daylight what until then had been visible only in an artificial twilight. Aside from the fact that the naïveté of the drawing recalled the sketches of cousins and governesses schoolboys draw, lovingly or mockingly, in their notebooks, M. de Pinamonte's formless masterpiece boasted an orgy of colors, clumsy and absurd to the point where I thought it outdid in its extravagance the most ridiculous imaginings of the daubers of Asiatic idols. No matter how unflattering the sudden rush of daylight was to the poor portrait, nonetheless I had to admit that it had not diminished the wonderful brilliance of the great, enchanting eyes. Once again I looked with love upon the divine mystery of that ancient sky scorched by unknown radiance; my soul again grew faint, abandoning itself to the perverse charms of those pupils, so large and fixed, so much so that it was with the utmost difficulty that I repressed the call of my heart, already on my lips, to the mirage of a long-buried passion. A breath as powerful as a strong wind of autumn, a whirlwind of old words and of names deader than dead leaves, rose up within me. Chasing away the mists of a false forgetfulness that concealed my own soul from my sight, it revealed to the eyes of memory the image of the ancient maritime city where I had the joy and the terror of knowing the incarnation of my happiness and my misfortune.

Pale with the hushed pallor of death, the silent water of the canals reflected the torpor of a city of deserted palaces and abandoned temples. A zephyr softly swung gardens of pensive vines on balconies flowered with rust, drowning in tarnished mirrors the yellowing train of their fairy robes. A stillness more unreal than the buzzing in a fever victim's ears hung over the entire city like the finale of a dream melody. The young and joyous city that I had loved had died with my heart's youth and joy. I recognized the ducal palace where the regent of S—— had introduced me to the gentlest of beauties: ruined doors, the broken steps of the staircase invaded by ravaging lichens, the entrances drowned in the green water of the *rii,** the high indifferent windows glistening with the poison colors of a rainbow burned by ancient suns. In vain did I interrogate the four horizons: silence, twilight, and oblivion had established themselves everywhere as absolute masters.

The noise of a footstep broke the spell of the evocation at the very moment when I abandoned myself completely to the strange perversity that impels us to search among past griefs for the cause of present trouble.

"Upon my soul, chevalier, the discontentment clearly marked on your face absolves me from making any excuse. I owed you some apology for my overlong absence, but I certainly will not make any for the sudden interruption of your colloquy with Manto. I have some right to be jealous of the beautiful sorceress; besides, I feared to leave you alone with her too long, for the lady is dangerous, even in a painting . . . And you, inflexible servants of a decayed house," the wag continued, turning toward the dejected mummies bent beneath their burden of tables and chairs, "you venerable scoundrels still faithful to the spirit of yesteryear and therefore superior to the powerful ones of our century, see that your extremely illustrious guest is served in the manner of the days of the true Brettinoros, and fly away afterward as if the golden age of whippings was not in danger of dying away forever."

As soon as the table was laid, the count-duke invited me to sit down, and we attacked with heartiness a most appetizing collation of coffee, toast, and preserves.

"By the Devil, chevalier, you are going to hear an account of an adventure which, contrary to my penchant for boring confessions, I have been able to keep absolutely secret until today. The sorceress whom you see here was its cruel heroine, and I who tell it blush to have been its ridiculous and wretched victim. I have had the honor of knowing you for barely a few hours, yet every little thing about you reveals the confidant whom my painful discretion has been awaiting for years. I want to open my heart to you—a poor heart indeed, by the

Brettinoros!—as simply as possible, and in return I hope for no more than a particle of indulgence for a story of which anyone but you would no doubt disapprove, both for its old-fashioned sentimentality and its salacious and ingenuous romanticism."

At this point the count-duke paused for a time, during which he coughed affectedly, blew his nose frantically, and spat dreamily in the direction of the enchanted portrait.

I looked with ever-increasing surprise at the bizarre narrator. The irrational old fool had amused himself by putting on over his suit a voluminous rustling robe the color of ox-blood, which emphasized shockingly the unnatural pallor of his face. A velvet cap very like the headgear of a fairground macaque, a pair of flowered and over-gilded Levantine slippers, the loose, dusty gloves of a former cardinal, and, finally, a handkerchief of Armenian silk, damp from the snuff-taker's sneezes, completed my host's peculiar outfit. M. de Pinamonte's attitude betrayed the anguish of a storyteller who, evoking some drama from the past, is secretly astonished at having been its hero. Deep, uneven lines worried the stormy, stubborn face of my Shrovetide masquer; and a small tear, lost in the raveled fabric of his wrinkles, trembled piteously like a dewdrop caught in the sinister trap of an ancient desiccated spider.

"Chevalier, do you know Venice the Beautiful, the Tender, the Unique? By Cain! The only excuse for that question is that it comes from the most brainless of men. Oh yes, you know the city of unsurpassed dreams and abominable awakenings. I'd wager that your visits there were as deliciously tormented as mine, and that your memories of it are as colored by melancholy as the confidences which you are about to hear. I have always adored the artificial animation and febrile gaiety of that dying, extravagant city. There love hides its face beneath a mask, and there the taste for adventure willingly cloaks itself in mystery, for vice, madness, and decay fear the light of day. No matter how curious my adventures may seem, the simple fact of their having had the Queen of the Adriatic as a theater will make them less boring or laughable in your eyes. Every country and every city has its own spiritual atmosphere, and nothing is more easily influenced by ambiance than the way we think and act. Thus I congratulate my adventure on having been a Venetian romance, for if it had happened to me in a country less propitious to fantasy, nothing would seem less urgent to me today, to tell you the truth, than recounting it to you.

"There is little to say about my life. My childhood was without love; my youth did not taste the sweet fruits of passion; and on the threshold of old age, maturity had come and gone without leaving a memory of friendship. My only preoccupation had been to fill, in a thousand extravagant ways, the place left empty in my heart by love; for the places where tenderness disdains to enter are visited by the scourges of lies, insanity, and horror. Even my sensuality had never been anything but a disorder of the imagination. For a long time my bitter, unhappy blood had carried the filth of Rome and the ashes of Sodom. Cruelly deceived in my search for pure love, I avenged my soul by polluting my body. The shame of my lewdness flowed over the child's flesh as the disgusting slime of October's snails drips from the flower. Wherever there was some hope of finding love, I sought it; and I remained alone in the midst of a blind and deaf mob. Nevertheless, I had, like all travelers, a thousand vulgar adventures of the Court, the coach, and the inn.

"I have read greed, stupidity, and hypocrisy in the most beautiful eyes of Europe. My heart was empty, my soul withered. I had never had any courage but that of debasement; with the exception of vice, I was timidity itself. I trembled at speaking to girls whom I later abused as brutally and as unnaturally as possible. Dreams of ambition had never bothered me; I was incapable of imagining happiness, glory, or greatness outside of love. Having very little gift for order, and also being careless of business matters, I shuttled incessantly between dissipation and stinginess, thinking to compensate for the former by the latter; whoever had known me as a spendthrift on Friday was amazed to find me a skinflint on Sunday. My melancholy had always been deep; the fleeting moments chilled my heart.

"One of the saddest results of the precedence which we accord to reason is that it turns us away from the profound sentiment of eternal things, thereby abandoning us to the agony engendered by our completely false idea of time. Is there a worse aberration than measuring the divine by means of the length of our steps in this world? What then is an accommodation between the need for adoration and the idea of the end? What, finally, is a past love or a future love? The difficulty of truly loving what is human has created a possibility of doubting universal love; our ephemeral attachments, poisoned by lies, have taught us to look for boundaries to the limitless Saana* of Tenderness, and in that way we have made a reality of time and turned love into a dream. Such weakness of mind! Such vulgarity of heart! We have learned to do without genuine love. Now, to live without love is to vegetate in ignorance of the eternal and, at the very heart of the most beautiful and passionate reality, to meditate stupidly upon the sacrilegious lament of time, of joy too brief and adversity too long. The chosen creatures of love, masters of eternal things, we have made our puissant life into two sterile, sullen parts, using one to kill the present and the other to mourn the past. That is why creatures destined for the exultation of love reach the edge of the tomb having known nothing but boredom and regret during their preparatory term on earth.

"Let me elaborate a little, chevalier, upon the miseries which were considered too rarely, in my opinion. Besides, I flatter myself that I know very well whereof I speak, for I have never met a wretch in Bedlam itself who could boast of having suffered as much as I. In other words, my life has been nothing but a long sickness of the tree of time, one of those mushrooms harder than stone that make a lump of mold on the tender weeping willows befriended by the moon and water. Outside of love, there is no cure for this diabolical affliction; unfortunately, my love met me too late and was never able to tear out of my marrow the voracious, aching root of my insanity. I was the cleverest of destroyers of hope, and at the same time the sincerest of creators of regret; in my eyes, that which is has no other reason for being than to cease to exist one day, the sooner the better, in order to provide my soul with an occasion to pity itself.

"Everywhere I went, the splendor of life burst forth like those great aloes, drunk with heat, which point the arrows of their belligerent flowers toward the sun; sea and sky met at my feet as time binds itself to time in the cry of love; on the bank of eternity powerful bodies twisted in the sun, sweet tragic bodies, bodies immortal as numbers or rhythms, whose moans of desire resembled the cry of some tremendous mystical dread; the entire earth presented itself to my view as an overladen wedding-night table—only the bridegroom was missing. And Pinamonte passed by furtively, his mouth twisted with false ironies, his heart devoured by the gall of distrust. Instead of seeking immortal love in gardens filled with flowers, sun, and voices, I directed my tedious course to the gloomiest regions of the world: toward the decomposing forests of the Baltic lands; toward the provincial cities of wild, unhappy Poland; toward small English ports, stagnant and crepuscular; toward certain old and empty Italian villages without past and without future; toward the mournful suburbs of London and Paris; toward . . . alas, chevalier! toward all the places degraded by the falsehood of unhappiness, ugliness, and death; toward every sinister corner where one is astonished not to discover the grave of some friend lost from view for years. . . .

"I leave the colorful square where shining fountains diffuse their coolness, where children dance in a ring in the misty afternoon sun, and turn into a malodorous, turbulent alley shivering with frozen shadows turning blue. I sigh, 'By heaven and hell! how empty is life, how long is time!' Everywhere I look are peeling walls, windows stained by rain or the rainbows of the past century; chimneys crowned by sour, sluggish smoke smelling of human flesh mixed with scaly grease. A heaven of shirts waves over my head—sad, pestilential laundry, the white of leprosy, the blue of epilepsy, and the yellow of diarrhea, urine, or jaundice—clothes empty of the hanged but full of drowned vermin. . . .

"I go forward among a swarm of thin, deformed children. Some of them are using dishwater to clean their poor feet covered with encrusted filth; others are delousing themselves as baboons do; farther away, in the shadow of doorways, behind the piles of broken boxes and empty casks, little girls reveal to their playmates the titillating, dirty secrets of precocious flesh.

"My heart and my thoughts remote from this scene and from myself, I continue my strange stroll through a nightmare of misery and ugliness, abominations, and excrement. Then my attention is captured by a sunbeam that illuminates a column or threshold of a church. I stop at once and gaze at the old stone warmed by the light of the past; the ghost of 'that which might have been and which has not been' appears in the hoary sun and looks for a long, long time into the glittering point of my eyes. 'I am she whom you loved in centuries past, in the time without name,' murmurs the pure phantom. 'I am she who once trod the same steps, to the sound of the same bells, in the time which is lost forever. . . . The daughter gentled by the fountains, high grasses, and shady places of the duchy of Brettinoro; the sister of your adolescence! The same steps, the same bells. In defiance of death, disgust, and despair! The city was so joyful then, do you remember? Proud horses, the grand carriages of the last century, the pale silks, the nebulous fragrances. And the loves in our souls, sweet as the mirrors of time departed, mysterious as the scent of water lilies, warm and pure as a cow's moist, soft muzzle! I am dead, O Sassolo, O Sinibaldo! I died when time died. The world will crumble, the stars will be extinguished, the memory of these ages will be obliterated in its turn; and I, I shall never come back alive; you will never see my flesh, you will never drink of its voluptuousness or of its tears. Happiness is dead; all is dust, all is ashes. What are you doing there all alone, shadow of yourself in the middle of a ruined city? What are you doing there, Guidoguerra? Who pities you, who loves you, who waits for you? I am dead and you are alone, horribly alone. Is it the courage to die that you lack? Who waits for you at home? Solitude, the ugliness of things, a long insomnia? Alas! time has consumed everything; time is more patient than the worm and longer than the tomb. Everything has been destroyed; only time is matter; only time is God.'

"The voice grows weak, fades, vanishes. A vast silence descends on my heart. I look to the right, to the left; no one. The first lamps are lighted; it is the peaceful hour of the bread and soup of poverty. Alone, Pinamonte! Here you are alone in the midst of a strange city, alone, all alone, far from everyone and from yourself, for the self is unknown to those who lack love.

"Come on, you old vagabond legs, forward! Come on, old bones, old feet, old shadow on the muddy pavement! Temple doorways do not welcome us; what we need is the silence and murk of stinking, slimy little corners of decaying blind alleys. . . . There, to the right, is the place where we can wait for time to end—and my gaze fell with love, chevalier, upon a fetid corner.

"Ha, Pinamonte, beggar of love, here is the filthy, moldy tomb you require. Sit down on that heap of old vegetables and sweepings, between those two groups of children, and glue your back, petrified like a reptile's, to the scabrous wall! Breathe deeply the pestilential air of this night which does not promise any tomorrow! Here you are, ordure in the midst of ordure, excrement among excrements! May the window of some hovel now open, and may a chamber pot empty its benediction upon your mad disputatious head, and it will be the fitting coronation of your accomplishments and your destiny. Ha, legs that have known intrigues of alley and court, here is a shelter for the night. Let time pass, let it die; we look for nothing more. Love is dead; only Time is matter, Time alone is reality. Let us sleep, let us sleep peacefully in the sewer of generations, faithful image of a world hostile to Love. Let us await the end of time, my soul, and after our death may ordure pile upon us, and may that be our tomb, our oblivion, and our eternity.

"How many nights of this kind are lodged in my memory! How many nights of being solitary, abandoned! I even recall awakening once lying in filth under a drizzle, half-strangled by a huge devil of a watchman in his cups . . . Ah, chevalier, I am painting a strange portrait of myself for you! To finish it with a few rapid strokes, allow me to add this detail: I was what is called imaginative, I had some knowledge of literature, I was adept at poetry; yet at the center of my harmonies I could perceive no voice that resembled passion's accents. Some of my verses were rich in music, others in color, but all of them lacked the tumultuous beating of the wings of love. In brief, never have I been anything but a mediocrity embellished with some eccentricity; and when you add to my hatred of untruth and my disgust with the world the intolerable contempt in which I held my own character, you will surely know the principal traits of my moral nature at the time of my adventure.

"I was then in my forty-fifth year. My soul embittered by mournful memories of the stormiest of childhoods, my body enervated by the insipid excesses of a youth only half-consoled by unclean pleasures for the loss of the illusions of art and love; prematurely aged by the incessant conflict in my heart between hatred of the human race and fear of solitude, I had resolved to end my days by going to some glorious, decayed city whose atmosphere matched my own decline—and, naturally, my choice was the marvelous capital of the Veneto.

"I arrived in that city toward the end of October. The sudden feeling of calm that came over me at the sight of the dreaming palaces and the somnolent waters seemed to be a very good omen for my dark lycanthropic plans. A peaceful, old-fashioned retreat, an artificial nostalgia for a historic past, earlier than the one whose memory torments us; and, finally, the company of a few serious books and of a humble, faithful soul—I know of no other remedies for melancholy. Quite proud of putting into effect my heroic resolution, I spent several days visiting the places dear to my youth, and afterward went to knock at the door of an ancient house hidden in the darkest part of a certain Calle Barozzi, whose sinister aspect I had noticed during a previous stay in Venice. I particularly liked the dilapidated house for the expression of sulkiness and hostility I read in its barred, dusty windows. I introduced myself to the queer, hunchbacked old woman who owned it. Giovanni's cunning eloquence did not fail to make an impression on madame Gualdrada; the witch rented me her lair for an extremely modest sum, with the exception of her own apartment of two or three remote rooms in the attic. I moved into my gloomy hermitage at once with the firm resolve never to leave it for any place on earth except that reserved for the dead. Alas, I underestimated the weakness of my heart.

"For six months I enjoyed the dangerous delights of reclusion and misanthropy, dividing my leisure—or, rather, my melancholy idleness—between the emptiness of metaphysics and the nothingness of my artistic or literary essays, when one evening, enticed by a soft breath of the gentle April breeze, I succumbed to the temptations of the outside world. With the faithful Giovanni I descended into the dim, quiet alley of which I had become an invisible inhabitant.

"Scarcely had I taken a few steps on the crumbling pavement when suddenly I saw emerging from the street of the Scuola dei Fabbri the grotesque figure of Prince Serge Labounoff, an old companion in debauchery at the time when I was swaggering about the court of the Semiramis of the North.* Foolishly, one drunken night, I had taken a fancy to this clumsy fellow of no family and no talent, and often since had cursed the unfortunate coincidences which, during my brief career as a diplomat, had caused me to trip over him in London, in Hamburg, and in Paris. Too close to danger to dream of escaping, I resigned myself unhappily to heroism and kept on walking. The moment he saw me the exuberant, stout boyar threw his arms, plump as those of a Muscovite nurse, toward the sky repeatedly and in a thunderous voice hailed me by five or six of my names accompanied by as many oaths and spittings. After which, pressing me to his heart and moistening my cheeks with huge, drunken kisses, flaccid and noisy, he howled directly against my ear, 'Help, by Hercules and Labounoff, help! I am dying of love, dear Pinamonte! Ah, let us beware of spoiling the joy of such an encounter by vainly evoking a youth without charm! A plague upon bygone days! May age ravage them! Hurrah for the present—and for as long as possible, for I am dying of love and also of thirst!'

"I struggled desperately in the Scythian's embrace and consigned him to all the devils; however, I had to admit that the torturer had good reason to link his name with that of his favorite divinity, for his dwarfish gladiator's arm did not release me from its spirited embrace until after it had sat me down forcibly on the filthy bench of a public bordello where, willingly or not, I was obliged to lend an ear more deafened than attentive to the Barbarian's erotic divagations, while sipping strange liqueurs.

"'She is a magician, dear little Brettinoro; an enchantress, a Circe, a Manto,★ the charmer who has clipped my wings. She looks at me with the air of Cynthia★ who has strayed into the kingdom of the Undines,★ and my wretched soul takes flight, departs, flees I know not where, as if it were in a trance. Daughter of a strumpet! Do you see her running, hiding, then without warning reappearing here, there, somewhere else?' (And with a hairy hand covered with barbaric jewels, the prince designated a dark corner where drunken knaves were taking turns caressing the fleshy charms of a street wench.) 'She speaks. Silence! She speaks. Silence, wretch! Do you hear her, dearest Pinamonte? She speaks: French with an accent from across the Rhine, Italian with curious, husky Spanish intonations. She speaks, I tell you. And I? Ah, poor me! I remain mute as a tulip, I look at myself in the light of the mirror attached to the hood of my hunting dog and remain lovingly and stupidly silent. For words lose their meaning in the distant, nocturnal barcarole of her voice. Her age? She is not in her first youth—which for us means seventeen, eighteen, perhaps twenty. But never mind. No one can say who she is, much less where she comes from; she is a great enigma. Yet the doors of the most austere palaces open at her step as if by enchantment. Very beautiful? Perhaps. But above all delicious, exquisite, charming. And admired by all, wooed even by damsels. Widow of a Florentine gentleman? A Spanish lady born in Ireland? She affirms it, it is claimed; I want to believe it. Bah! An adventuress, you will say. So be it. Let us admit it. Nothing is surer. But what difference does that make, by Hercules and Labounoff? She came here five or six months ago, accompanied by her brother Alessandro, hardly older than she. A curious personage, I must say! A gentleman with the manners of an accomplished crooked gambler, but very pleasant, too pleasant perhaps, for his manner always reminds me of the mincing ways of the gentlemen with lace cuffs. But once again, let us pass over that. Despite the fact that the minx has taken a liking to me and seems to trust me completely, her slowness in rewarding my ardor would be the despair of anyone but the conqueror of Catherine. Now it makes me dote all the more upon the lovely child, the beautiful pigeon of a wench; and because I have no better friend in this world than you, I absolutely must introduce you to the charming object of my infatuation. You'll see her eyes. Her eyes! Do you recall our moonlit nights at Windsor? In the eyes of my goddess you will find once again your beloved mists spangled by the mystical moon, a moon mad with love. You must know her eyes. You must; I wish it. Ah, viper of a dove! Ah, too kind hussy!'

"I will not attempt to repeat the whole of the prince's besotted discourse, for that would plunge me into endless detail.

The eloquent passion of the gossipy tale continued far into the
night, and the only way I could halt it was by making a formal
promise to accompany my Muscovite to the gala being given
the next day by the old Duke of B—— for the beautiful Manto,
Countess (or pseudo-countess) of—by the Styx! the name es-
capes me. Besides, what do you care about her name, chevalier? Ah, I have it! Annalena de Sulmerre! Clarice-Annalena de
Mérone de Sulmerre!"

From the penetrating look the count-duke gave me as he
pronounced the name of the enchantress, I understood that he
had expected a movement of surprise on my part; however, I
had had a presentiment concerning this thorny passage of the
story and permitted no glimpse of the confusion into which the
adored syllables had thrown me. Unfortunately, the effect of the
impassivity that had cost me such great effort was exactly contrary to what I had logically expected; for this cruel M. de
Pinamonte, throwing himself back into his armchair and furiously waving his head, arms, and legs, suddenly burst forth in
impertinent peals of immoderate joy.

"Chevalier of my heart and of all the devils! The attention
that you courteously deign to accord to the babbling of an old
fool honors you, for I am perfectly aware how unlikely it is that
you will be entertained by the recital of an adventure that does
not concern you in any way!"

Although I had little taste for the Neapolitan's irony, light
as it was, I considered it the decent thing to conceal my annoy-
ance behind a vague smile, while the treacherous Pinamonte,
visibly amused by the bittersweet grimace of his victim, continued his account in these words:

"I should prefer to keep silent about the exceptional emotional state into which I was cast by the prince's importunate enthusiasm; for of all the despicable passions that burn in the hell of human blood, physical jealousy surely is the strangest and the most painful. Despite my efforts, I could not stifle the movements of my heart that the amorous ravings of my former companion in revels aroused. The portrait of his love the romantic boyard had delighted in painting for me bore a remarkable resemblance to the mirages whose gentle melancholy beauty I had spent my capricious youth pursuing in vain. Once again I trembled before the terrible emptiness of my destiny and, returning to my lonely, gloomy house at daybreak, I was consumed with both a cruel ardor whose object I did not know and a blind, ferocious jealousy whose cause I tried without success to understand.

"The obscure principle of this feeling, so far removed from the problems of reason, soon became the chief subject of my meditations; nonetheless, I was never able to identify its nature with certainty. For jealousy is closely associated with love, and love itself is hardly conceivable without a specific object. As difficult as the question was, it continued to illuminate for me certain aspects of our nature. I am indebted to it for the knowledge that most people are less attached to the reality of that which they love than to the illusion that connects the chosen creature to the innate image which they maintain in their own minds. Does there indeed exist a real lover who, in order to consider attentively the object of his tenderness, does not close his eyes to reality and turn his interior vision to the depths of his own soul? Ah, chevalier, we always love only one being! This unique creature we carry in the deepest part of our unconscious; it is identical with our destiny, with the eternity of love of which our soul is the indestructible home. Whoever loves truly loves God!

"The following day the prince did not fail to come for me at the agreed hour, and without lingering unduly over the libations which were customary during our meetings, we left the dim retreat of dreams and misanthropy by gondola for the palace of the old Duke of B——.

"The footman who announced us was dressed in scarlet livery. On the threshold of the light-flooded hall I let fall my right glove; the carpets were of a soft old rose color. I raised my eyes, and realized all at once that a new life had just commenced. I noticed a blonde lady at the center of a group of mature gentlemen, grave and decorated. A certain fountain dear to my adolescence, in the park of my ancestral home, began to sing in my memory; on the rim of its basin was a bench eroded by stiff, scorched mosses; the weeping willow's leaves brushed the yellowed old pages of my *Don Quixote de la Mancha*. Alas! Love was there! O joy! Time had ceased to exist! Someone pronounced my name, then that of the duke. Old di B—— still had a very precise recollection of my wild grandmother, the famous lady Guidoguerra. How little that rejuvenated us! A blonde woman dressed in old gold surrounded by a group of callow youths and solemn, decorated old men!

"A resurrection through love, a miracle of art: Eurydice herself singing an air by Gluck; an Athenian marble coming to life with the breath of an eclogue by André Chénier—certainly it would be beautiful, assuredly it would be sublime. However, it would still be art. Now, art is to life only what our existence itself is to the absolute of love which is reflected in it. I saw a blonde woman in the middle of a circle of stupid sycophants. It was life, to be laughed about, to be cried over, life, all of life! Her appearance was Poetry, her walk the Dance, her voice was Music. I recognized in her the sublime trinity of Movement. But she herself was much more than all that: she was Life, Adoration, Prayer. I recognized in her all the Callirhoë* of Fable, all the virgins of Judea and of Greece, all the women of the *Pensées,* all the Babylonian girls of the Court of Charles II, all the fairies of the forests of April, and . . . who knows what more? I immersed myself in the great, veiled eyes, I let myself be lulled by the pure, cool voice, I lost all sense of things. I was far, far away from life and far from myself. I found myself in an old enclosed garden, sick with a hazy vertigo of wild flowers. Evening was falling. In the distance, a maiden sang, sang for me alone, the canticle of life fulfilled. O grief! Lost forever! Proud, enigmatic, full of malice and tenderness, nostalgia and cruelty. Life, life itself, all the enchantment of living. It was Circe de Mérone, it was Manto de Sulmerre! The archangel of Sensuality! The demon of Dream, the very dream of adolescence. Ah, how horrible is a dream which comes true! My most secret wish had just been granted: before me was the shy child of the ancestral park of Brettinoro, the familiar phantom of my youth. . . .

"Alas, how deep the sadness of a wasted life; but the emptiness of destiny accomplished is deeper yet, for our hearts are made so that the place occupied by waiting can be filled only by disillusionment, and nothing can follow desire but something that resembles, whether on close examination or from a distance, satiety!

"However, my melancholy did not last long. Labounoff introduced me. I was surprised to hear, in the familiar syllables, a name which was almost strange. I was transported far from Venice and from myself. Of all rare surprises, perhaps the most precious is that of hearing from an enchanting mouth the simple, soft words we are expecting. Usually the mind, that bitter, sterile little thing composed of a dash of foolishness and a portion of wickedness—the mind, hideous embryo of the great human lie—poisons the most natural smiles. Why must it be that, at the first sound of the unknown voice, the beloved real face of Beauty, Truth, and Love transforms itself into a foul mug where all the ugliness of Suspicion, Slander, and Falsehood leers? Is it then so dreadful to permit a glimpse, under the painted sky of a ceiling, of what we once were beneath the real sky of the first day? Alas! When life's simplicity becomes difficult, life itself has long since been an incurable evil. Sulmerre, the great Fairy, the Lady-Child, opened her lips . . . surprise of surprises! Where, then, had I heard before this silence of water, sky, and plain in a single sound, in one indistinct first sound? In what Eden had I been greeted before with these simple, wise, primitive words: 'How glad I am to meet you at last! People spoke of you so much in Naples, in England, in Germany!' I could find nothing to answer; I am not at all a man of glib rejoinders, but remarkable names of distant isles, of fabulous lovers, of angels and books, flowers and constellations, crowded to my lips tumultuously, and my heart was like a leaf in the whirlwind of my heart. 'No, you will not fall on your knees sobbing in the midst of everyone! It would be truly absurd; think of the extreme ridicule. . .' Such were my thoughts, such were perhaps my first words—how do I know?—for I heard laughter around me.

"The Fairy was in front of me, the fairy of the park and the fountains, the fiancée of my childhood. I spoke. Someone spoke who was myself and whom I did not know. Past youth and lost days cried, cried deafeningly within me: 'Her eyes! Just look at her eyes, those enormous ancient eyes in which a night of horror, love, farewells, lies, and tenderness burns!' Someone spoke of voyages to far-off countries, of noble services rendered to King Poniatowski,* of adventures in Muscovy, Sweden, and Spain. . . . By the Styx, I was terribly eloquent! 'Yes, madame, in Seville . . . no, in Nuremberg. . . .'

"O you, you, my youth suddenly returned in its entirety! O you, you, laughing phantom of my childhood, show me your hands, assassins of small infatuated nightingales, your poor hands, your soft caressing deadly hands. You know, you know, how well you know; the large ponds at the bottom of the gardens beloved of autumn! And the bloody, frozen frogs that we fished out of the mute marshes in December, and the majordomo who recounted to us over and over Madame Guidoguerra's amorous escapade in a carriage all across the kingdom of Naples! And, in the center of the murmuring shrouded park, the little ruined pavilion full of rats, owls, and spiders . . . and the pleasant *Don Quixote* of Monsieur de Florian under the weeping willow, near the babbling fountain . . . O you restored, mine, miraculous! Sacred spirit of solitude, shadowy confidant of fairy retreats! It is you, really you, o small hands of a cruel friend, of an amorous sister, you and you only, strange, slender, swift hands of my dear mistress! You, and not the willow, not the evening breeze, you who turned the pages of the book with dilapidated engravings: Sancho finding his donkey again. Maritorne* the sleepwalker. The handsome captive Christian and the sweet wife of the sultan. The knight of the Mirrors. And de la Mancha on his pallet of agony. . . .

"I was alone then, o Manto, o my enchantress, and young, and I exhausted my soul in sterile, amorous transports, and I was dying of nostalgia, and you were only a dream. Gentle friend, so close to me now, so dreadful, so real. Circe walking dressed in my shadow. 'I know of certain adventures of yours, my lord. . . .'

"'But madame, these are only slanders, rumors noised about by fools . . .' I was so sure of pleasing! I changed colors, positions, intonations, and affectations with incredible rapidity. What had happened to my timidity, my distrust, my repugnance for living and speaking in the manner of the times? Who exactly was this Monsieur de Pinamonte, this stranger so full of arrogance, tenderness, and temerity? I completely abandoned myself to the intoxication of my verbiage; an unknown person spoke with my mouth and I joyously applauded remarks which would have made me blush at any other time.

"What was this? What the devil did it mean? Ah! it was no longer Venice, no longer the ducal palace of B———, no longer the vain appearance of life; it was life itself, the promised kingdom, the landscape of milk and honey of the country of Love. I no longer doubted, I did not know how to doubt; the whole of life was no more than an immense, profound, magnificent affirmation. I possessed my Manto; she was mine. I could not take my eyes away from the eyes of my dear angel. The flicker-

ing fire of their pupils fascinated me; in them I discovered reflections of unknown lights, extraordinarily distant glimmers that
seemed to emanate from the Atman★ of adepts. A mystic spring-
time bloomed in my soul in the rays of an adorable spiritual sun.

"O learned and delicate oddities of a Paracelsus,★ of a Nettesheim!★ What is life, if not the manifestation of the necessity to
adore that which already is God? What is life, if not the love of
love for itself? The blood of my ancestors had awakened in my
heart; I was knight, conqueror, troubadour, ambitious cardinal,
poisoner doge, hysterical pope. O moment of eternity, O wise
folly of love! It was the most frivolous of conversations with an
adventuress who would soon cause me grief of more than one
kind, and it was happening in a palace swarming with heraldic
vermin and scribbling rabble, alive and real. But by Cain in the
moon spots, the eyes, the dear eyes, the terrible huge eyes of
times past, of forever, of the hereafter!

"Wandering in the enchanted solitudes of these nostalgic
eyes, I felt like the soul of a child filled with wonder by a fairy
tale, or an amorous astrologer lost amid the lakes and mountains of some sleeping kingdom of the Galaxy. The fabulous
sky of the lady Sulmerre's eyes were not like the blue of any
stone, of any distant mountain, of any horizon of this world;
even less would I dare compare it to the azure of flowers or of
springs.

"Since my separation from la Mérone I thought on several
occasions that I had recognized it, that blue of ecstasy and sweetness, in the flickering of vaporous fires of certain essences, and
especially in the image preserved in my memory of perfumed
lamps. I looked into the eyes of the sorceress and thought of

the fire that, in my grandmother's story, drowsed together with
the Princess, the Courtiers, and the Chicken on the Spit. The
eyes of the adventuress were heavy with the past dreams of my
childhood and the future silence of my death; in interrogating
their mystery, I discovered the secret sense of that old exclamation that seems so trivial at first glance and so dear to lovers of
every variety in every age: 'Such or such a woman, such or such
art, such or such passion is *my life*.' Because all defined feelings,
all personified loves, are only manifest forms of a unique love,
an eternal love which is the principle of being.

"While talking of a thousand and one frivolous matters we
had unknowingly moved away from the others. You can imagine my surprise at finding myself *tête-à-tête* with Annalena, my
precious love, on an isolated terrace in the midst of the most
beautiful arrangement of statues and fragrant shrubs that I had
ever seen. My first emotion somewhat calmed, I thought it more
polite to moderate my eloquence and repress my desires. The
lady Mérone spoke: I was all ears. I gazed at her somber blue
eyes, I listened to the dear voice that was at the same time close
and far away; the pure bells of the departed months of Mary
sang in the sky of my childhood and my simplicity. Chevalier,
chevalier! what a ravishing conversation that was! 'Most assuredly, madame, I am delighted with the Duke's party.' . . . 'Is
our boyar a good friend of yours?' . . . 'What? For ten years?
In St. Petersburg? The rascal! Is it really possible?' . . . 'Odd, I
agree, but so gallant.' . . . 'Do brush off this powder . . . No,
no, you clumsy thing. This is a fashion that really has lasted long
enough!'

"I listened, I approved, I exclaimed. It was so true, so simple, so sweet! These were most ordinary things, of course, but that devil of a Pinamonte never noticed. Life was so young! The hour ahead was truly unknown. O surprise! So many antiquated, used, decayed things all at once made new! Blossoming of moments, freshness of eternal spring ceaselessly renewed!

"The remarks we exchanged differed very little, no doubt, from the usual conversations of polite society. Nevertheless, at each moment I discovered some unknown charm, some new significance. My defeated reason was dead, I had become entirely heart, a great liberated heart that palpitated from my knees to my brain. Each time I attempt to describe by means of a perceptive comparison the state of exaltation in which I found myself, my thoughts return to those born blind whom the Word of the God of Love suddenly flooded with light. I was full of surprise and, at the same time, an immense confidence grew in me, newer than any astonishment, mightier than any terror. My sight had just acquired the power of penetration. I raised my eyes and knew the universe of love, that boundless sky that only an hour ago was the shadowy field of my blindness. I contemplated the marvelous garden of space with the feeling of looking into the most profound, most secret part of myself; and I smiled, for never had I dreamed of being so pure, so great, so beautiful! A paean of thanks to the universe exploded in my soul. 'All those constellations are yours, they are in you; they have no reality apart from your love! Alas! how terrible the world appears to him who does not know himself! When you felt alone and abandoned before the sea, think what must have been the solitude of the waters in the night, and the solitude of the night in the endless universe! How you have suffered, and what suffering you have caused! O man, O man! What is the pain of darkness to one struck by blindness!'

"Then I looked again at Clarice-Annalena, and at once my intoxicated soul continued: 'See, she is beautiful and she is life! Do not scorn her, do not ask too much of her, for she does not know what she gives. Hold her tenderly, look at her lovingly, speak to her gently, examine nothing. For she is life, and she knows not who she is. True love is unique, and will soon find itself alone face to face with itself. She, she is only life: cherish her, for its moments are counted. Rush to love her, for it is growing late in the world's day. Forget who she is: she has eyes, a mouth, a voice, a sex; she is love's creature, the creature of your love. If you judge her, you shall be judged. If you love her, you shall be loved. If you abandon her, love will hide its face and you will return to the impossible void. Nothing in her is impure, for her master is the master of this night, this instant, and of your tenderness. Is she a little liar? Is she a contradiction? Love has come, love has healed, love has saved.'

"The newness of my feeling became drunk with the youth of everything. The mysterious charm of the hour and the agreeable solitude of the place could but hasten the first outpouring of a love-struck soul. We were surrounded by the most exotic plants of Asia and Africa; the harmonious constellations of spring shone with a gentle radiance above our heads; the beguiling whisperings of universal love mingled with the sighs of the breeze and the water's gurgling. 'Do you not have a thousand thanks to offer me,' resumed the mysterious spirit of nature itself; 'Have not your most secret wishes been granted? Have not the Blessed Isles floated to meet the confident navigator? Do you not know

now that, of all lands, Atlantis is the closest? O fortunate mortal, you have conquered your grief and your sensual pleasures, your joy and your melancholy!'

"The moon shone very high in the heavens; the sky, the earth and my spirit became intoxicated with its strange brightness as from a wine of eternity and love. Sublime and grievous beauty of imperfect things! Melancholy and joy, voluptuousness and pain! She had enjoyed the most sinful loves, she whom I would have wished to know bathed in the radiance of virginity! The broken wings of my archangel dragged in the mire of life's blood and tears. A swarm of frightful salamanders stirred the ashes of her past; the queen of my destiny, chevalier, the queen of my destiny was a strumpet!

"A disturbing smile hovered upon Annalena's lips. In all four corners of an adjoining gallery stood discreet old love seats. I drew Mérone to my heart, threw her down savagely and took her in an unimaginable position with delight, sadness, and disgust. Fragments of distant serenades reached us at intervals on the zephyr's wing.

"Whatever it was that happened, my life began again. Yes, chevalier! I, Pinamonte, I, Brettinoro, lived the hours, the days, the months. Swift hours, perfect days, ephemeral months! And I was loved—oh, yes, by a strange whim of fate—loved with the best and the worst love. To be, or even merely to believe oneself, sincerely loved by a fallen woman, wanton of the fields, girl of the streets, or intruder in palaces, is perhaps what remains of the most curious, the richest in joy and pain, the most contaminated by compassion in this miserable life.

"I was neither young nor handsome, yet my fanciful person was not without some charm. La Mérone's melancholy was equal to my own; she belonged to the category of women who are more attracted by the ugliness of a cultivated lover than by the handsomeness of a vulgar fop. Our natural propensities matched wonderfully. On top of that I was Brettinoro, Benedetto, and Guidoguerra, and the remains of my patrimony permitted me still to cut a respectable figure in society. In short, I could believe in the sincerity of la Mérone without worrying too much about appearing ridiculous.

"Soon nothing was talked about in the palaces of Venice other than the fancy that the Countess of Sulmerre had taken to me. Our names were on all lips. I had become the assiduous guest of an ark of dreams anchored in the torpor of the Riva dell'Olio. The hours chimed; sounds of oars approached, moved away, died. It was day, then night, in the dim high windows of the past. I knew all the inebriations of love and all the torments of jealousy. Now life was there, so close to me, and time no longer existed, and this vanished time devoured my life. Voracious passion swallowed up my hours, my days.

"I loved. I was jealous of my own body, of the unconsciousness of swoons, of the memory of sensual pleasures unconfessed, unknown, forgotten, of the possibility of unfulfilled betrayals. I made lists of suspicions and of revenges. I hated Annalena's breath, I cursed the life of my unique one. I would have liked to enter living into the closed paradise of her dreams, into the distrustful hell of her thoughts, her desires, her recollections. I sank into bottomless meditations on the secret meaning of her movements, the inflections of her voice, her perfumes. I groveled before her most despicable, most bestial attitudes; coldly I analyzed the taste of her hair, tears, sex. I madly searched the horizon beyond her eyes. Sometimes I heard, among the moans of her lust, the supreme Name, the stammering of the Absolute! My hands grew thin, my eyes became strangers, mirrors clouded over at the sight of me, doors creaked my story to each other in the twilight. Then . . . then the enchantress fell asleep with her head on my knees, my reason forgot everything, and my soul dissolved in the seventh heaven of joy.

"These cruel cares were often joined by the belated and somewhat ridiculous regret of having supplanted Labounoff. To tell the truth, I had always held my so-called friendship for the prince in little regard; however, nothing in this world is more tyrannical than a feeling compounded of compassion and scorn. Although perfectly aware of my relations with Annalena, he never indicated it, showing no trace of a vexation that anyone else in his place would have displayed. He did not even consider it necessary to interrupt his assiduous attentions. I met him at my mistress's home very frequently, and his sincere haste in taking leave of her, approaching me with a laughing air as soon as I appeared, sustained me in the thought that he had not taken his misfortune too much to heart, or else that he was pleased, in accordance with the Slavic precept, to sacrifice love to friendship.

"As far as making any allusion to our love affair, there was only one instance and that under very strange circumstances. On one particular day as I wandered in my stupid melancholy through the popular quarters of Venice, I was surprised to recognize a carriage with the boyar's coat of arms at the entrance to the winding Calle Selle Rampani. I entered the narrow alley

with the most indifferent air that I could assume, and soon saw
my Muscovite supported on one side by Alessandro Mérone and
on the other by one of the *moujiks* of his retinue. A swarm of
urchins and small children swirled around this bizarre group. His
lordship's visage seemed to glow more than usual; his elation
gushed forth in foul terms; wig askew, sword between his legs,
he advanced haltingly, meanwhile brandishing with a disconcerting fury the bodice of the beauty he had just left. My first
thought was to follow my usual course by allowing my long
legs to carry me away, but the accursed tippler had already seen
me and, what surprised me even more, recognized and hailed
me with thirty-six oaths. I was obliged to put a good face on it;
saluting the pest with my most hypocritical smile and without
stopping to deliberate even for an instant, I launched myself
despairingly into the rumbling abyss of his breast. 'By Hercules
and Labounoff,' cried the ruffian, pressing my head between his
thick hands as if it were a cluster of grapes, 'By this starry sky'—
it was the hottest time of the day—'yes, by this luminous Orion
and this bright Bear which loom above our heads! By all the
trouble which Christopher brought back from the New World,
I swear that my heart is free of all malice and that never has
resentment entered my soul. So, Pinamonte, innocent dove!
What madness of yours is this to avoid me—what am I saying?—
to run away from me as you do? You are loved, traitor? You
are happy, torturer? A fine affair, indeed! These are the pleasures and triumphs of your youth.' (The sadist flattered me.) 'I
love, understand me well, I love, I worship in you the favorite
of fortune and of love. This was my own destiny; for, between
us, was it not the whim of my noble mistress . . . Enough.

Alessandro, insensitive soul, cold heart! Kiss at once the dear friend of the beauty of beauties! Kiss him at once, dog, if you want to save your life. All of you rogues, from the biggest to the smallest, from the handsomest to the ugliest, kiss him! And, failing love, may at least a little salaciousness come to gladden my soul! Come! Come to my heart, my handsome Sandro, my brigand, my little orphan! Come! Let us swear to be at the perpetual service of the count-duke in his love affairs, to help him with all of our might!' (Zounds, did they help me later on!) 'I am dying of thirst, Sandro, Sandrinetto! You, Basil, Ivan, Plato! Bring me something to drink at once, or I shall ravish your mothers! . . . Ah, my young pigeon, my celestial Pinamonte, you are cruelly mistaken about me. And how little you know the heart of a Slav! Give me your hand. A plague on these little doves of beggars . . . The roses of my life are faded,' he continued in a hoarse voice punctuated by belches and hiccoughs, 'My head is the color of winter.' (And his wig was flying toward the sky.) 'I have no more passions than those of a grandfather. To hide myself behind a wall, to bounce on my knee a baby boy and his little sister, this is all that I love, this is all that comforts me. For I am a poet in my own way, Monsieur de Brettinoro, and, unhappily for me, I have a very sensitive heart.'

"At this moment a fountain of vomit gushed from the gargoyle's thick lips. Alessandro and his companions grabbed him roughly and pushed him into his carriage, and immediately, dumping the filth from the gilded windows, the heavy coach was driven off headlong in a great din by a disheveled, merry *moujik.*

"As ridiculous as this encounter was, it soon became the

subject of new torments for my anxious mind. I began to analyze in a thousand different ways the sentimental drunkard's remarks; I became entangled in endless considerations of the way I had behaved with him; and, finally, I accused myself stupidly of treachery and cowardice! For egotism and love were so intertwined in my feelings that it was no longer possible for me to discern if I was the insensitive slave of one or the faithful servant of the other.

"One of the benefits of my love was to reconcile me with people. An unknown force—a pleasant, gentle force!—led me at the end of a beautiful day to colorful, tumultuous Piazza San Marco. With innocent heedlessness, I thrust myself into a sea of ruffians, Levantines, dandies, lackeys, procuresses, wenches, flower sellers, vendors of candied fruit impaled on a stick like frogs, adventurers of every nationality, urchins of every age, and pigeons of every color. Heavens! What infamy, what lies, what disgust! How the old viper quivered in my breast, but how cool were the devoted lips of love on the inflamed bite! I was full of astonishment, anger, and desire. When will it come, the promised day, the day of all days when the solitary being will feel himself moved to his very depths before a crowd of men as he is at the sight of the sea or of a forest? Why is it that oceans of trees and of waves unite in a revealing song of love, while a hundred human beings brought together are enough to create the most absurd, the most hateful of monsters? O peaceful herds! Slow-moving white rivers at the foot of hills! How much closer you are to the heart of God! O docile harmony of great migratory flights in the mistiest of ocean skies, what spirit of order and of beauty inspires you! Vile, cruel beings, stench of creation!

When there are just three of us, Love is still among us, but when we are thirty, the authority of an earthly master imposes itself immediately. And when we are one hundred thousand our name is State and our life abomination. Fierce suffering and cowardliness below, insolence and cruelty above: the father become tyrant, the disciple inquisitor, the warrior instrument of lies, pride, and rapacity; and there, at the very bottom, the enormous, the unknown, the obscure, the undefined created from the sob of a prostitute and the swoon of a virgin; from the coins tossed onto the money-changer's table and the death rattle of a hanged man; from the glint of a sword and the cry of childbirth!

"Wait a moment! I suddenly caught myself, laughing; no, no, three times no, friend Pinamonte! Your anger and your sadness no longer are timely. And don't let me catch you bragging again, hypocrite! Tell me, what is this little fury that is overcome by a great desire to laugh? Is it really today's humanity that is repugnant to you? Isn't it, rather, yesterday's humanity! Bah! Pinamonte, a light little being in the morning breeze, adorable creature of May, carefree and dancing, a great hunger for love has awoken in your entrails; look, judge, weigh—the monster of your life is before you, all lies, all ugliness. Swallow it! Infinite wisdom has measured it against your hunger; swallow it, I tell you, swallow it now! Go ahead, don't be afraid, you will digest it. What? No sooner said than done? Your disgust! Really? Your disgust! A fine thing! Know that there is only one disgust, one alone—that of our impotence in attacking, in conquering, in devouring, in digesting the great enemy hidden inside ourselves. But times have changed; you have attacked, you have vanquished, you dance on the deflated corpse of your vain and foolish weakness; you love yourself, you think and you speak the truth, you are the lover of man!

"Thus, driven wild by wisdom, I parted the massive human wave, blending with the tremendous canticle of the universe the small sharp sound of my hypocritical sniggering. Soon I was loving this exciting odor of flowers and of filth exhaled by our amazing mob; I even got used to the madness of arrogance and mendacity. These things will soon be over, I said in my heart, they will end when it will please the great Love that they should end. He knows what remains to be done, he feels what remains to be done, he does what remains to be done. This absurd rabble is filled with unconscious tenderness; let us love it. Was it not condemned yesterday, will it not disappear tomorrow? Let us love, let us become intoxicated! He, He alone remains; here He is; He comes; the stone of Jerusalem glows in his hand!

"I continued thus; my shadow, like that of an anxious heron, soon developed a fondness for the pavement of the Piazzetta, the columns of the ducal palace, and the refreshing paving stones of San Marco. My attention was drawn by the clever nonsense of sycophants. First my purse disappeared, followed soon by some small ornaments; this only made me laugh. Misfortune to fools and daydreamers, I repeated by way of consolation. Several times I spoke to pretty girls with beauty spots. My watch disappeared like a dream, my snuffbox vanished like a light mist; even the gold buttons of my jacket were torn off with great gentleness.

"Nevertheless I continued my sentimental promenades like an imbecile. Things inspired an intense curiosity in me; soon my tenderness for Venice equaled my love for Annalena. The

Woman and the City fused into a single being in my mind. Besides, are there two things in the world better made to understand each other and to fuse together than divine passion and archangelical Venice? Who then, stopping on the Ponte della Paglia on a moonlit night, would not be overcome by this consoling and sublime verity that for the lover of Beauty there is no dream without a corresponding reality?

"And who could have contemplated the pale, sleeping *rii,* the pure palaces like orphans, and the great, all-powerful dazzling Molo without recognizing in these fraternal things the melancholy of his tenderness, the thrill of his memory, and the tragic sun of his love?

"Velvet bench for the knees of prayer, palace of amber, myrrh, and azure of tenderness, Venice is also the precious repository of tears of all amorous human grief, and the heaven which reflects the paleness of last hours and the prostrate immobility of separations.

"Here savage nostalgia illumines with its tears the face of ignominy and the eyes of cruelty itself; and when the floating Isola di San Giorgio is outlined in the black of death against the purple of the wind, and when the storm rumbles over the unsteady city, it is hideous Shylock, suffocating with love and hate, who in the evening calls to Jessica who is gone. And this Venice whose soul is torn, this former ruler in her finery of queen of carnival, is also a winsome Venice, feline, cooing; and whoever loves to flirt with melancholy or to tickle grief like a girl also enjoys the falsehood of affecting a rose costume and a flower tied by its stem to the handle of his sword while strolling in leprous, romantic alleys. And this Venice perfumed with the spices of the Levant also is a kind of Rome emasculated by the worship of saints rather than of God; and when the bells sound the blue-gray song of evening like sweet-throated communicants of bygone days they remind us in their singular way that long ago it pleased our master Love to be born of a little virgin, most humble and most adorable. And this Venice sick with love is also the sister of languorous and disquieting saints; and when the gold of a waxing moon gently falls on the shoulder of a leaning tower, you think of Mary Magdalene breathless under the weight of the urn of holy perfumes.

"Too noble to be a courtesan, too graceful to be a mother, Venice the Bewitching is a lover and only a lover; so beautiful that she makes one cry, she knows also the power of old pagan charms, and it pleases her to reign over our hearts by mystery as much as by grace. Powerful as Venus, like Venus she was born from the sea, thus proving once and for all time that every symbol has flesh, every dream its reality. And as she feels, our supreme creation, that nothing can be more precious to the God of love than this mirror of beauty and tenderness that man humbly holds out to him in his weary hands torn by stone and by metal, as she feels this, she, breathing product of our hands, contemplates with confidence the splendor of eternal things and tenderly sighs: O heavens, o seas! And you, days, and you, nights! Indestructible flesh of universal love! I, mortal, fearful and gasping, I the created one, I am your equal in saintliness!

"Thus Pinamonte awoke one morning in love with two beauties at the same time! As a nickname I gave my sweet one the delicious name of the city, and gave the city the suave name of my beloved. All that was in my heart, all my sentimental trea-

sure of heartaches and joys derived from the great Dogesse of
passionate stone and of magical water; it was easy for me to escape the denigrators sheltered in her breast, and to convince la
Mérone to follow me; nevertheless, I succumbed to the super-
stitious fear of separating my precious twins and of snatching
the flower of passion from the intoxicating hothouse where I
had watched it bloom.

"One day, strolling under the veiled gaze of the thousand
windows of the square, I suddenly felt the eyes of Love upon
me and bowed my head respectfully. O beauty! O potent silken
rose, offered by Love to Love! O beauty, God adoring himself!
Could you be anything other than a mystical sign in your slightest
manifestations? My heart filled with a delicious anguish; I walked
toward the palace, great delicate flower of a thousand doubled
stems, and as I embraced passionately one of the lower columns,
the pulsing of human blood merged with the heartbeat of the
stone inflamed with love. For love, chevalier, love resides in the
heart of stones, and it is with a poor pebble, infused with tenderness and picked up on a solitary shore, that the teeth of Falsehood and of Arrogance will be smashed on the day of days.

"It was my unfortunate fate that Labounoff surprised me
one evening at Santa Maria della Salute as I was humbly kissing
the dust of the paving stones. My sweet secret was revealed; the
entire city mocked me unmercifully. I looked at those who were
laughing and I laughed louder. What could be more amusing,
in effect, than the spectacle of a stone saturated with love, and
of a fool mocked by the little devil Arouët!*

"Another time when I was plunged in some passionate and
preposterous meditation, I remained motionless for a good

---

couple of hours in front of a pharmaceutical window display: sunlight played on the charming colors of the various potions, and the devil whispered to me with the voice of the apothecary that what I saw before me was the Riva degli Schiavoni set ablaze by a magnificent sunset: 'How close you are at this moment to the sweet, ravishing mysteries! Love has regenerated you, healed and saved you; passion has made you the confidant of nature, my dear Pinamonte! How much you love things! How much things love you! All this splendor spread out before your eyes is the product of Love; and this eternal and sublime Love is complete in you. What am I saying? Are you not yourself this powerful love, this eternal creator? This rapturous, shimmering Venice, is it not a lover's dream, your dream of the eternal lover? Ah, Pinamonte, I prostrate myself before your power; I deliver up to you Hell; you have triumphed, Creator! Before your footsteps the dark wing of the Contradictor drags in the dust. You have won, Love! Falsehood is finished, it exists no more! Now there is the sublime harmony of the first day.'

"With that, I awoke from my ecstasy, chevalier of my heart, and went on my way with ten or fifteen crowns' worth of drugs in my pockets. In order to rid myself of these chemicals I found nothing more ingenious than to sprinkle them over the sweepings at the foot of a wall; and this brought about another of the most beautiful miracles of Love by upsetting, by means of the gentle splendors of his youngest city, the stomachs of all the cats of the parish of Santa Maria Zobenigo!

"Sometimes my restless, jealous spirit gave me a respite of days or even weeks, when a somnolent indifference replaced it and I felt myself become the Pinamonte of old, the man disillusioned by worldly things and, above all, convinced of how little he could count on human friendship or love; in congratulating myself on what seemed to me a return to reason, however, I misjudged in a strange way the nature of these peaceful interludes, for they were in no way a sign of recovery. The too-brief respite they accorded my anguish ended without fail in some mad, hideous emotional crisis, sometimes taking on the aspect of the most repugnant sentimentality. Thus I could not gaze upon the sumptuous fabrics or the dazzling gems with which my Manto was covered without immediately crying out plaintively: 'Annalena's poor little dresses! Her sad little jewels!' I lost myself in ludicrous, touching attempts to restrain my sighs and defer my tears when my mistress broke a piece of bread.

"Three times a day our table was laden with exquisite, perfectly composed dishes, and my dear minx customarily attacked them with the sharp teeth of a famished wolf cub; no doubt the charming zest with which she nourished the body of a young woman in love would have been an unceasing delight to a rational suitor. Nevertheless, this great lump Pinamonte, accustomed as he was from long experience to discover objects of pity in the merriest spectacles, as a rule received nothing from Annalena's splendid appetite but the saddest impressions. 'Pitiful creature,' I murmured, 'pitiful creature exposed to the whims of fate, to the rigors of climate, to the failings of poor human nature! Here you are in front of me, weak, fearful, ephemeral! You are nourished by the fruits of earth fertilized by death; you eat with sadness and only to maintain today's melancholy until tomorrow's afflictions. Alas, too much like the cannibal who in his fond cruelty fattens his captives before handing them over to the kitchen executioner, the tomb nourishes you with its fruits so that tomorrow it may find a more abundant treat in your round throat, your succulent arms, your substantial rump! O abandoned creature! So pitiful, so ridiculous in your sovereign beauty! I look at you. What are you doing? You carry to your lips a glass of old smoky wine. What? Is the chill of death circulating already in your veins? . . .' And a thousand other such absurdities of the same kind, chevalier, for from the beginning until the end of our remarkable repasts *tête-à-tête,* I never ceased to complain in this fashion.

"The view from a prison refectory or from a hospital surely would have affected me less than the daily sight of this beautiful gourmande, her youthful vigor diminished by naughty behavior, gaily reviving herself with copious mouthfuls drowned by long glassfuls. My terrible heart sometimes went so far as to be moved to pity for my strumpet's shadow, the unhappy shadow condemned to lie on the cruel marble paving stones, or to run into the sides of fireplaces, or to sweep the rugs of the Levant!

"Sometimes I would wake my dear Annalena more than ten times in the course of a single night in order to reassure myself that she was not dead. The movement of the clocks filled me with dread, the fleeing moments made me tremble; I looked for silver threads in the sweet hair fragrant with youth; and when the saucy girl mocked my lunacy I sighed idiotically: 'Unlucky one! Unlucky Annalena! Only another hour until old age, only one more day and it will be time for death! Cold, blind, pitiless death!'

"In the natural flow of my thoughts this funereal vision of an old and sickly Annalena became linked to the image of my own deterioration. That in turn led me to a comparison of age and vital force, and the double disproportion I discovered was a clear reminder that the rapid decline of a man in his forties would spare me the pain of witnessing the decline of a girl hardly more than a child. . . . Nonetheless, the nervous love of the last Brettinoro hardly derived any satisfaction from these delightful calculations. In true passion, the discovery of a distraction from some anguish is rarely anything more than a simple substitution of one worry for another. The idea of being the first to be struck down by the decrees of Time quieted my uneasiness regarding Clarice, only to make me shudder all the more for myself. What a ghastly thing for a lover is the approach of an age that dispels illusions and makes the body unfit for love! How I hated the excesses of my youth! How I cursed the blindness that had caused me to waste the treasures of passion in debauchery!

"Sometimes I woke with a start in the middle of the night and its silence with the strange feeling of having outlived the earth and the sun. I would light the candle and run to the mirror; the image that my gaze saw there filled my spirit with terror and disgust. Heavens! those lusterless eyes, that careworn forehead, that contrite air, that pallid and grimacing long face of an old man! Could this be the tangible form of a soul sanctified by love? O terror! O despair! The wavering flame of the torch, whether I held it close to the cruel mirror or moved it away, made my ugliness flicker in the glass; clouded or clear, the truth that emerged from those depths made me shudder! With hate and sadness, I examined myself meticulously and, aside from a certain air of oddness and grandeur, discovered only gloom and repugnance. 'Certainly,' I sighed, 'nothing can equal the beauty of an impassioned soul that purifies the object of its love; but look at that long nose between those cheeks of old fruit harvested by the wind! And while nothing is greater than a spirit which, searching for love, discovers God, how happy, how triply blessed are young, strong, well-shaped legs!'

"If I turned my back on this impertinent mirage, the frightful phantom thumbed its nose at me from every corner of the dark hall. If I closed my eyes, the Double grimaced at me from the deepest shadows like a victim of drowning. As one might expect, I spoke to no one of these ridiculous terrors and especially did not let Annalena suspect them; my beautiful one could not help but notice, however, the surpassing joy which her compliments on my face or my appearance gave me. I noticed that truly young and truly graceful gallants normally paid slight attention to praise of this sort, and I resolved to model my behavior after theirs in similar circumstances.

"It happened often also that after the intoxication of sensual pleasures a crushing lassitude swooped down on my soul, a disgust without reason, a sadness without limits. I would look at the silent Annalena curled up in the dull light of a high window, open upon an eternity of *ennui,* and sigh: 'Ah, my poor little thing, how white you are! White with all the whiteness of insipidity! How the devil could I have delighted in you a moment ago? Please—do me the favor of closing those legs of a nervous little girl: your slightly sour intimate odor makes me ill. Instead, show me . . . no! don't show me anything, not even that which under my stern hand makes a sound so childish, so fleshy, and so hot. Nothing, nothing, for you have reverted to the purely organic. Remarkable little device, odorous and complicated little machine. . . . I could hardly stand your reflection in a mirror of rose water. What are you doing there with just one hand offered to my sight? Ah! die, and let the blind vermin of life fatten ignobly on all this tepid white pudding of love!'

"Poor Clarice bowed her head and, like a beaten little girl, gazed at a faded flower in the carpet; then, hiding her face in her long orphan's hands, she began to snivel bitterly. 'Oh yes,' I thought then, 'this is the old story of Colin and his shepherdess, of Hortense the baker ill-treated by the king's soldier. A story of eternity, a story of the moment. What could be more natural? Ingratitude at the smell of old boots, squeamishness at the nauseating vapors of swaddling clothes.' I grabbed my hat, kicked the door, and descended the staircase on my backside, spitting the vapid bile of my disgust right and left. As soon as I reached the street I hailed a gondolier and had myself taken as quickly as possible to my lodgings so that I might deplore with Giovanni the destitution of my soul and the cruelty of my heart. I reach my house, and what is the first object to greet my sight? Annalena, my dear chevalier! The beautiful Mérone, the gentle Sulmerre, the indulgent, the merciful, who was able to precede me in my demented flight and who greets me on the very threshold of my melancholy retreat with a smile, a kiss, and a tear. The young, the exquisite Annalena, very white and very tall, in the cloak of a female doge on the doorstep of my dreadful crumbling house! Ah! By the Devil, by all the Devils piled up in the hell of a human soul! All is forgotten! I kiss the sister, I kneel before the lover, I drag toward the dusty depths of my darkest recesses the image, both human and divine, of love. O lost woman, found again! O lover! Come, let me press you against my old, half-dead heart! Let me lay on your soft mortal body all the weight of a philosopher's cadaver! Come, love! Let the immense night of voluptuous delight roll over us like an ocean, and let us be like the drowned tossed up at random by the waves!—One more kiss, and then let us separate, sweet separation, mysterious, fearful, veiled, and masked. And let no one—not even Giovanni—see you as you flee like a gazelle.

"A last look, a last laugh. The tender Sulmerre left me in the most clandestine way in the world. . . . Here I am alone, drunk with happiness rediscovered, alone, all alone and joyful in my shabby hovel in the Calle Barozzi.—And tell me, chevalier: what do you see me doing now, now that la Sulmerre is returning happily to her chiseled palace of the Sleeping Beauty?—You see me busy playing now the dog, now the jackal, biting the carpets with a savage joy, overturning the furniture with the enthusiasm of an epileptic; sticking out my tongue, preening in front of the mirrors. My wig flies in the air, my watch dies under my heel; my chest resonates like a forge under my furious fist; I am here and I am there; I jump like a jerboa* and fall back a toad; I run, I skip, I leap, I slither. Here I am naked, here I am dressed again; I laugh and I curse; I exult, I twitch, I explode, I am bathed in sweat. Annalena came running, Annalena forgave, Annalena understood, Annalena trembled, Annalena loves! What better proof of love than to dash as she did from her palace to my ruin— in a carriage, it is true, but isn't it a quarter of a league all the same? A quarter of a league! Imagine that, chevalier! What goodness! What sacrifice! In truth! And here am I finally on the Ponte

San Maurizio, my old friend, speaking of my happiness to the ancient house on the corner, to the gloomy house with huge doors and vile green shutters, its doorsteps awash. . . . This ancient, deserted house, taciturn confidant of my simple-minded raptures and my insane despairs!

"Such were my joys, such were my sorrows. La Sulmerre was the source of a feeling that no one but she in the entire world inspired. The mere sight of her was enough to give rise to the strangest movements of my soul. I no longer lived except in her; sun and flowers, breezes and water, woods and echo, silence and shade were all Annalena, all Clarice. There was no contour of the adored shape that did not recall some amorous vision of my childhood or of my youth. La Sulmerre's movements, the inflections of her voice, the nuances of her gaze stirred in my mind strangely distant associations. Often I contemplated her as one looks into one's own profoundest depths. To a stranger who one evening asked me who this beautiful lady was, I answered distractedly: 'The initiatrix.' I spoke sometimes to my charmer of these peculiarities; she smiled at them, and I laughed at them like a maniac, for every passion has its divine hours and its earthly moments.

"I arrived at the sublime and perilous state of mind in which one identifies the loved object with love. Each day I became more detached from my own identity; away from la Mérone I felt less than half of a person, and to see her again after a brief absence was to find myself once more, to return to my flesh and my spirit, to be reborn. On moonlit nights I took her by gondola to the Lido. Her presence united the most hopelessly remote worlds and transformed them into objects close at hand.

I showed her a star, then another: 'Here is Yesterday,' I said, 'and here is Tomorrow! The infinite radiates the sublime confidence of Love!' And I spoke the truth; my heart shared the great passionate calm of nature. What did it matter to me that my affection had feared the judgment of men? I was not afraid to look into the very depths of the eyes of Eternity, and my feeling of divine security triumphed over both the sadness provoked by my lover's past and the uneasiness inspired by the dubiousness of her present state. Could I indeed condemn as vain and sterile an attachment that had succeeded in restoring me to love and to life? There is no such thing as barren passion, for the love that does not increase is a love that revives.

"Annalena was my whole life, and I could not bear that any object whatsoever of which I was fond should remain unknown to her. How sweet I found it to speak to my beloved of the poor, solitary old things that I loved! With what feeling and astonishment and pride I introduced the ravishing creature to those things I loved! Toward evening I led her to the old bridges dear to my reveries; I showed her the ancient houses my fantasy enjoyed peopling with fabulous Sinibaldos and dream Clarices. I introduced her to lethargic banks, to obscure, ruined corners, like a young lover presenting his new bride to his circle of relatives and friends.

"One evening, under the sinister entrance to the Ghetto, I spoke to her of Shylock and of Jessica; to my great surprise the great barbarian genius who had shocked me so by his oddness suddenly revealed himself to my Latin soul in all his beauty, all his power! I reread *A Midsummer Night's Dream, King Lear.* Then I went back to the tenderest, the strangest, the most blessed:

I reread *Julie,* the *Confessions.* What! I said to myself, this Shakespeare, this Rousseau! have they then never held a pebble in their hands? Really! How was it that these great lovers of Nature did not fathom the amorous principle of their Immortal One? Being so simple and so strong, why did they not know or not dare to follow their sublime feelings to the end, to establish the supreme Being and to recognize Him, Him, Him completely, in their human love? I gave the first part of the *Confessions* to Manto. Our shared feeling for the Genevan strengthened the bonds of our friendship.

"One evening we went into San Maurizio. The church was deserted. A great terror rose in my blood. I seized the beloved hands: 'It is the Epiphany, the Epiphany! On your knees, Clarice! For he is here, He, He the Father in the boundless heavens, Son on the circumscribed earth, Spirit of Truth, love of the Father for the Son, love of the Son for the Father, love of Love! Love, unique, confronting itself! On your knees, on your knees! For it is there, terrible in its mercy, before our Gentile eyes!'

"What more can I tell you, chevalier, of the extraordinary state of my heart? How can I describe it to you with profane words? I am not a saint, and even at the height of my amorous exaltation I was far from being in a state of grace. Alas! No, the rain was not my sister, the wind was not my brother; but I said to the wind: 'Gentle brother of Clarice,' and I said to the rain: 'Tender sister of Annalena!' The things most different from youth and beauty, objects the most remote from love, reminded me constantly of my beauty, my lover. Separated from her gentle image, nature and life lost their significance. Did I happen to leaf through some ancient folio in an out-of-the-way bookstall?

The perfume of its moldiness made me think of an Annalena in the finery of olden days, of a Clarice of times past.

"One day I came across a most remarkable book: *The Holy Year Practices of Friar Martial of Le Mans,* penitent monk. Immediately I developed a passion for this celestial work. Admittedly I blushed at my unworthiness, but I noted that the love of a creature taught me to adore the Creator, the Father of all things. I sometimes said to my lovely, in the most serious way in the world, 'What, dear face! Will this wintry weather never end? Why do you not want to bring the spring?'; or else, 'I'm tired of sleeping, my sweet one; please deign to say, "Let it be light!'; or again, 'There's something I'd like to say to or ask of my friend Stanislas.* Order His Majesty to appear at once!' My precious love clapped her hands, her laughter pealing forth; I ended by laughing myself. Nevertheless, my soul remained serious; love, divine love, and trust in love remained graven in the depths of my soul. For I saw in my Clarice a personification of all-powerful Nature whose essence is Love; my Annalena was to me like a reflection of the Revelation. I recognized in her my tenderness and my joy as well as my sorrow and my pity; yes, her love taught me to pity youth and beauty as well as joy and sensuality. 'May pity be my only wisdom; may my perfect love of creation be my love of God!' My whole body was invaded by my heart, a heart throbbing with amorous pity.

"Nevertheless, I continued to have hours of doubt and despondency for, although accustomed to the fluctuations caused by my hypochondria, I was still somewhat surprised by my fits of febrile, unconsidered commiseration. Even as I abandoned myself to the strange vagaries of my nature, I sought to penetrate the mystery of this striking compassion for a creature upon whom destiny had lavished its most precious gifts. Reflecting upon this subject shattered for a time my burning exaltation. The loves of human beings, chevalier, are commingled with distrust, fear, and contempt, and what we call pity is only, in most cases, our contempt for that which we love. We know too well the meaning of our pity for our own kind not to fear being pitied in our turn. Astarte and Asmodeus* still are the princes of our pitiful friendship. Contempt poisons our compassion just as the desire for punishment corrupts our concern for justice, for, just between us, nothing could be farther from the love of virtue than the sinister and pusillanimous ardor with which we seek to eliminate from society whatever we believe endangers its dubious harmony. The position of magistrate is to a certain extent merely a tribute we pay to the prince of this world, to the father of deception: the jailer and the executioner would satisfy ideal justice for most of us. For, not content with being more ferocious than the tiger, craftier than the fox, and more venomous than the serpent, we have been able to add to these bestial advantages that purely human virtue, the spirit of vengeance. Once past thirty years of age, the majority of human beings live only in order to avenge themselves. We avenge ourselves of the harm that is done to us, and we avenge ourselves also of the good that we do; there you have the reason that our life so strongly resembles a pile of filth soaked in blood. Love, forgetting faults, pity! All the possible grandeur, all the actual baseness of man! Let your mind dwell for a moment on the admirable and terrible mystery of pure feeling, and you will have a perfect vision of the ghastly barbarousness in whose shadows we live completely surrounded after eighteen centuries of Christian effort. Alas! how long must we wait for the return of Him who will communicate to the weak, the sad, to those deformed in spirit and in flesh, a little of his glorious mercy, of strength and joy and beauty itself? When shall we learn to feel sorry for Joy and for Beauty?

"Thus I sometimes questioned my compassion, but the love of love never left me. Nothing in the world concerned me except my affection. I loved Annalena even to the profound mystery shrouding her past. I knew nothing of her life other than some affairs of the heart which she had confided in me at the beginning of our liaison. As to the rest, her care in keeping it secret equaled the caution of her brother Alessandro. Neither the delicate feeling that led her at such a tender age to cultivate the arts, nor the wisdom which she demonstrated in the midst of such singular circumstances, nor, finally, the air of propriety that she was able to assume in her quite exceptional situation, none of these qualities of heart and mind astonished me as much as the contrast between the heedlessness displayed in her confessions about past loves and the skill with which she eluded any question that might relate to her birth, her parents, or her early years. Moreover, the proof that I gave her of my natural and somewhat brutal jealousy doubtless was of no help in encouraging any effusions. At the beginning, such reserve on a subject that was bound to arouse tender curiosity was a source of continuous vexation; however, I soon became accustomed to the mystery surrounding my strange happiness, and finally even found in it a charm of the most troubling sort. For one and the same law rules both our adoration of God and our love of man; blind abandonment to feeling and wise submission to the unknown share equally in both, and we never love better than when we ill understand, because the impossibility of acquiring a thing with the coin of reason reminds us of the marvelous treasure of feelings that we carry in our hearts.

"After several weeks of suspicion and sulkiness, the subtle affinity between mystery and love revealed itself to my mind in all the charm of its sadness. I was grateful to la Mérone for having remained a bit of a stranger even while abandoning herself to me with a lover's beauty and a sister's tenderness. The duration of earthly loves is measured by the melancholy concealed beneath the joys they give us, for the pleasure of being aware of the so-called reality of things is little compared to the sublime pain of not knowing how these things will end. I let my gaze wander often over my naked dreamer as over a charming landscape on a May evening; I interrogated the great silence of her eyes more beautiful than the sleep of the waters of summer; I became intoxicated with the somnolent perfumes emanating from the wild garden of her hair; I slaked my thirst at the cool and pebbly fountain of her mouth; I inhaled the sweet-sour wine of her young carnality as the Scythian drinks the sap directly from the willow's wound. Nevertheless, the most secret possessions did not succeed in satisfying my mystic desire. 'Here you are, close to me, here you are very close to me, here you are below me, at last, like the mountain under the cloud, like wheat under the rain, like the rock under the wave; and here am I in you, now, like wine in the vessel, like the heat in the fruit, like life in the blood. And here we are united, now, like the bell and its sound, like God and love, like pain and pleasure. And here you are already a little farther away from me, and now farther still, and here we are separated by a dark abyss. O woman! what creature are you? O Clarice, what lover are you! Your destiny is as alien to me as your sex; I know nothing of your existence in the universe, I know little of your life in time. Whence do you come? Who are you? Where are you going? Azure atom in space, tiny drop of dark water in the luminous ocean of Love! How terrible it is, and how sweet, to be a stranger to that which one loves! Let others suffer torments because of their ignorance of the superterrestrial sense of their love; I am pleased to know nothing of mine, nothing, not even its effective existence. No, not the present nor the past nor the future! O sure shape of my life, O bread and wine of my passion, how I rejoice not to hear your true name! Love brought you one evening, death will carry you away one day; such was and such will also be the fate of my own flesh. The body is alien to life, the coffin alien to the corpse. I know nothing of myself; should I seek to understand your secret? Let us stay as we are; all goes splendidly; let us become drunk with the mystery of the moment! Let it suffice to know that love is in us and around us and in all things, that there is not a pebble which is not completely suffused with it, and no sun which does not receive its light, because whosoever seems to shine with his own light shines with the light of love. Let us remain in peace. Its reign will come to pass. Its name will be sanctified!' This was my evening prayer. The malicious Annalena sometimes responded to it with an innocently mocking *amen,* after which I stretched out my long, argumentative cadaver alongside my dear life, she whose breath was strong and sweet.

"Quite often in the course of my nocturnal promenades my whimsical reveries took me back to the past. The moon spoke to me of the insomniac nights of my childhood, of the grounds of Brettinoro and the fountain within them, of the songs of the old nurse who loved the fountain. The lulling aroma of the water recounted the endless history of my wanderings. The wind spoke to me of a thousand distant lands glimpsed in bygone days and long since become once again foreign to my heart, for man has a truly vivid recollection only of those places where his soul loved. 'Your springtimes are already legion, monsieur de Pinamonte.'—'Peace, peace, O my cruel heart!'—'You are old, monsieur de Pinamonte,' insisted the melancholy mischievousness of my heart. Oh yes, by the pitchfork and the tail of the Devil! I was old, I knew it; what need was there to keep reminding me of it? 'Ah! Lean on the railing of the Ponte Ca' di Dio and look into the farthest reaches of the night! It suits you well, to tell the truth, to play at indifference . . . That's it, one hand on your sword hilt, the other on your hip; you look delightful. Straighten your peruke, please . . . Ah! the dandy, the ridiculous gallant, the fickle one! Don't expect me to believe that! Hear me, I know you, we know each other, I am your heart, your poor old simpleton of a heart. You have suffered much, monsieur de Pinamonte. But also the agreeable rage of loving nothing in this world! Can one be happy without loving oneself, I ask you? And can one love oneself when one loves no one?' I blushed, I swore like a devil, and I never succeeded in silencing my villainous regret; completely ashamed, I ended by agreeing with the mocking, featherless old bird of my conscience. How much my past seemed to me empty, frozen, miserable! The sky was pure, Venice slept; a great emotion throbbed in the wind. 'You haven't loved, you didn't know how to love! And now love descends upon your old age, ardent as a reproach, terrible as revenge! Now you know it!' Oh yes, I knew it! A new being cried out with love in the darkest recesses of my being; I was filled with joy and my joy was pain; I was filled with pain and my pain was more beautiful than my joy. My love sought in vain expression in my mind, in poetry; only in the Scriptures did it find a voice, and I sang with David:

O God, thou art my God; early will I seek thee: my soul thirsteth for thee, my flesh longeth for thee in a dry and thirsty land, where no water is.

To see thy power and thy glory, so as I have seen thee in the sanctuary.

Because thy loving-kindness is better than life, my lips shall praise thee.

Thus will I bless thee while I live: I will lift up my hands in thy name.

My soul shall be satisfied as with marrow and fatness; and my mouth shall praise thee with joyful lips.

When I remember thee upon my bed, and meditate on thee in the night watches.

Because thou hast been my help, therefore in the shadow of thy wings will I rejoice.

My soul followeth hard after thee: thy right hand upholdeth me. But those that seek my soul, to destroy it, shall go into the lower parts of the earth.

They shall fall by the sword: they shall be a portion

for foxes. But the king shall rejoice in God; every one that sweareth by him shall glory: but the mouth of them that speak lies shall be stopped.

"And, while arguing with myself, I continued my erratic course through the sleeping streets. Yes, by heaven, my heart was right: I was ridiculous. . . . My attenuated and desolate shadow moved over canals, pavement, and walls. It was ludicrous. My sword's shadow attached itself to my shadow like the tail of a disillusioned baboon. Scrawny and stooped and split in two, the shadow of precocious old age! I was old, but—by the Styx!—what did I care about the insult of time, the emptiness of life elapsed, the treason of memory? I loved; I loved the dear, the detestable Mérone. I adored; I adored the dear, the detestable Pinamonte. I had discovered finally, belatedly, a reason to live, that is, to love myself. Sometimes I caught myself kissing the reflection of my face in mirrors; having been caressed by the hands, the lips, or the tears of Annalena, my visage appeared to me divinely beautiful and as if illumined by a heavenly sweetness. I looked at my body—this poor emaciated body of an aging fop—and bowed low to myself like a pagan in front of his idol, for I felt that my flesh was in some way hallowed by the pleasures it had been able to give the divine Sulmerre.

"My mistress sometimes enjoyed speaking to me of the oddities of my bearing, of my face, and of my character. I too discovered every day some lovable detail of the vampirish ugliness of my friend Pinamonte. I was barely accustomed to my happiness; my solitude had left me so abruptly! Now this argumentative madman, this gentle demon, had a place to lay his

71

dessicated old head. . . . A cushion of sweetness, of dreams, and of illusions waited there for me in the old house of the Riva dell'Olio: la Mérone's breast, the bosom of la Mérone, all warmth and softness and oblivion. What gesture would she make, the beloved, upon seeing me enter her boudoir? Would she be gently reproachful on the subject of my somnambulist adventures? Would she sulk? Ah, if only she would deign to be the least bit suspicious of my virtue, to show me a little jealous vexation! What would be my joy, what would be my triumph! I studied the extravagant contours of my shadow on the stained-glass window, shifting in the moonlight, I arranged myself in various ways: with the air of a Prince Charming, with satanic affectations . . . Yes, that's it, there: I wish to appear shortly before my beautiful one with a nonchalant air and smile on my lips. I shall surprise her seated on her cushions deep in some pernicious book. I wrinkle my clothes and my jabot, I half unbutton my jacket, I hunch over and give myself the appearance of a thoroughly bad lot. Now I am ready to make my entrance. I advance on tiptoe, like a thief or a suitor. A mischievous smile plays upon my lips. I enter. I hear her little cry of surprise: 'Where the devil are you coming from at such an hour?' I stammer anything at all while giving a little cough; I pretend to avoid her gaze. She orders me to look her in the eyes. My reply is ready: 'No more playacting, my most beautiful one; what! would you dare to suspect me. . . .' I do not finish. 'Ah! the traitor, the ingrate! In what condition does he come to see me! Cruel lover! Your silence is a confession, a confession of treachery! Don't come near me, barbarian! Don't come near me! Heavenly powers! When will you put an end to my torment?' I can stand it no longer, chevalier of my heart; I run to throw myself at the feet of my dearest, I cover her with kisses, I drench her with tears; I press my beloved wildly to my heart, I admit my flirtatious guile, I tenderly kiss her entire body, I cradle her, gently I rock her to sleep in my arms. . . . A saintly odor of sensuality bathes the bedroom; each new hour seems to bring a new silence. From time to time a cricket utters a little plaintive cry; a piece of furniture creaks. . . . la Mérone sleeps against my heart; sleep overtakes me in turn; I fall asleep in the arms of bliss.

"With such dreams, monsieur le chevalier, with such nonsense was my mind occupied. There was not an event, a thought, or a word that I did not relate to la Mérone and which did not seem connected to my love. In my eyes I had become the center of the universe; I perceived the most secret meaning of all things; my miserable heart, saturated with bitterness, now beat in time with the divine harmony of the spheres; the circulation of my amorous blood intoxicated me as if with the music of inexhaustible water-clocks. Passion initiated me into the mysteries of being; my love for myself was the love with which the divine burns for the divine.

"In this way I lost myself in the strangest daydreams until the moment when, opening my eyes to the heavens, I realized that time, implacable time, had not interrupted its course. Waking myself then from my foolish reverie, I leaped in the air like a devil, then was off like a shot. Anguish bore me aloft like a flying machine, and surely it must have been highly amusing to watch me rush headlong to the place where my gallant duties awaited me.

"I arrive at the threshold of my earthly paradise; trembling,

I open slightly the door of the sanctuary. . . . Alas! why must reality have so little resemblance to dreams? O my childish dream, o my precious desire, where are you? Where is the lamp, where is the French novel which arrived with the latest mail, where, finally, is la Mérone herself? I enter and see only shadows; I proceed, I listen . . . nothing moves . . . I hear only the peaceful, regular breath of the sleeping woman. Alas! assassin of dreams! Bitch of reality! La Sulmerre did not find it opportune to wait for me; la Sulmerre does not love me. Cursed imagination! You tricked me with your hollow mirages of love and tenderness and sincerity! 'So, is it you, monsieur the somnambulist! It is most salutary to take some fresh air before going to bed. . . . Come, come to me . . . I can't wait to recite the introit,* and in an hour or two we will begin singing matins.'* Sombre and silent as a dead man, I take off my clothes, I lie down next to the dear hussy and, consumed by the aphrodisiacs of frustration and disgust, I begin to make love to her savagely. When I awake, Phoebus already is high in the sky and I feel quite playful. Do I not have la Mérone near me? Does she not love me in her own way? What more do I need? Is not this the goal of all human beings? 'Good morning, dear monsieur! Such a beautiful sun, such a charming day! Ah! by the way! Haven't you invited the prince and several other friends for this afternoon?' Such is life, monsieur le chevalier, such are our loves, and this is how the world is.

"This, however, was the philosophy of my best days or of the heaviest hours of lassitude or resignation. Most of the time the slightest indecision in Annalena's look and the faintest hesitation in her voice were sufficient to change my mood abruptly.

Then the torments of jealousy and rage followed the tortures of anguish and pity. I was suspicious of all forms of what is foolishly called 'possession': none of them was able to satisfy my demented desire. My raging passion subjected my dearest one to the cruelest practices of depravity, the most hideous forms of obscenity. I took horrible pleasure in separating myself, in metamorphosing myself in my imagination; in my mind I took on the gross form and the strange features of a drunken sailor, of a soldier hot with the blood of rapes and massacres, of a senile, drooling libertine eaten away by aphrodisiacs. I was at the same time actor and spectator in my tragic ignominies. I disguised my dear mistress as a strumpet, I made her up as an appalling, saucy old tart; I dragged my love to brothels, I bathed my dear archangel in latrines. By pushing her, by persecuting her with dreadful prayers and wild threats, I forced confessions from my dearest one that made me tremble with fury, shame, and lust: I had myself initiated into the frightful mysteries of her old loves and, not content with being jealous of my own flesh and of all the living, I incessantly reminded myself of those former lovers, and multiplied their number to infinity. I went even farther; thanks to the intimate details revealed to me by Annalena in her transports, I penetrated the soul and the flesh of my predecessors and played, a mime struck by madness, the drama of their passions extinguished long ago, the comedy of their hopes deceived, the farce of their lost joys; and when my shameless art tore from Manto's swooning lips the name of the lover whose playful or fierce lust I mimicked, a ghastly feeling of disgust and triumph harrowed my soul and shook my miserable flesh. Demoniacal, I was possessed by a legion of rivals.

"Among all these admirers, departed, forgotten, or betrayed, whose enumeration undoubtedly would appear pointless to you—diplomats, prelates, renowned actors, swordsmen of all countries—only one seems to me to be worthy of mentioning, particularly because of the curious phenomenon of feeling that he aroused in my heart. He was a young Dane of the highest quality. . . .

"During one particular night of insomnia, as I combed through an old armoire I found by chance a melancholy portrait of the forsaken one. The fickle Annalena told me the story of this gallant in words so full of tenderness that I suspected her immediately of still harboring some love for his memory. However, the once-cherished name of the Scandinavian had vanished from her frivolous memory, and the only name I ever knew for this gentleman was the ridiculous nickname of Benjamin that the little monkey had thought it amusing to attach to him. The face of the young man, shining with nobility and sweetness; certain traits of mind and character; the subject of his separation from la Mérone; the original turn of phrase of his farewell letter in which he informed the ungrateful woman of his desperate departure for China; and last, the rotten trick that the perfidious one dared to play on the unfortunate fledgling in making known to him through Alessandro the news, as cruel as it was false, of her death and her burial in the cemetery of Vercelli— all these strange details of her story were as so many eloquent pleadings, earning the unique sentimental worshipper of my Sulmerre the indulgence and compassion of a madly jealous lover filled with repugnance for the vulgar, transitory fancies of other rivals.

"Benjamin's unhappy love offered me an excellent opportunity to enter into Annalena's heart and mind. From the way in which she related the story, I judged that among the Dane's numerous qualities, she had appreciated only those which, in her eyes made him appear a timid child, affectionate and easy to dupe. It was clear to me as well that what she took to be inexperience and ingenuousness was only a very conscious need in me to maintain my late-blooming flame by creating as many illusions as possible about her. The slave's cringing craftiness, the courtesan's pitiful hypocrisy, the mother's triumphant tenderness, how well I knew all of you through studying the character of la Mérone! The surprise she showed at seeing me so full of commiseration for Benjamin made me clearly aware that she had expected from her confidences only a fresh outburst of jealousy on my part. No matter how strange my sympathy for this unlucky gentleman had appeared to her initially, she lost no time in discerning it to be an indirect proof of the profound love of which she knew herself the object. She spoke to me naively of her discovery; I pretended to be astonished only by her perspicacity; in reality, the weakness of my own heart surprised me much more than my lover's acuteness. Oh yes—what I loved in Benjamin was the love with which he had burned! I was grateful to him for having been consumed with grief and care for a creature who had ignited the cruelest fires in my own heart. After all, was there anything so astonishing in that? Tenderness is more clear-sighted than the wisest experience, more fertile than a June night, and more delicate than the architecture of swallows. All is wisdom, mystery, and sweetness at the heart of profound love, of the pure flower of God stupidly soiled by the vile, hideous human lie. Benjamin had suffered, Benjamin had loved; the love and pain with which my heart overflowed loved the gentle Benjamin as the couple lost in the night loves the star that smiles at them, the breeze that caresses them, the silence that hears their tender whispering. I had become used to considering the young Dane as a kind of secret companion of my misfortune, an invisible witness of my happiness, the ideal confidant of my troubles. Thinking that I would never meet him apparently encouraged me to confidence. Sometimes I would sigh: 'What can our friend Benjamin be doing? Is he still in Formosa? Has he rediscovered an interest in living? The poor man! If only he had someone close to him who knew how to console him! Such sorrow, Annalena, such sorrow!' La Sulmerre pretended to share my tender feelings, but I think that she was more affected by the distress of the speaker than by the misfortunes of the absent one. Woman is made thus, monsieur le chevalier; it is inconceivable to her that one could live in the past; her flesh, her heart, and her mind recognize time only in the present moment, like the dragonfly and the rippling of water. And the great future open to men who love and to animals is closed to her.

Despite the fact that the sly creature appeared often to hark back to the time of her love affair with Benjamin, I always had some doubt about the sincerity of her regrets and strongly suspected her of encouraging my pity only to expose the generosity of my feelings. Women are weak and the hypocrisy of weakness is unfathomable. Not content with having found from the beginning an excellent proof of my love in the esteem in which I held the Dane, the deceitful thing soon turned it into a means of defense, which she fell into the habit of using on the slightest pretext. If a rather strong word escaped my lips, la Mérone boasted at once of the moderate speech and honorable ways of her sentimental admirer; if I happened to reproach her coquetry or to suspect her outright of infidelity, there followed a hymn of praise to the sublime trust that Benjamin had never ceased to demonstrate the entire time they had known each other. 'So, dear Allobroge,* is it a pastime worthy of Your Lordship to torment ceaselessly a poor heart without malice, an unhappy defenseless girl? Insensitive man! Corrupt heart! So you have taken it upon yourself to avenge my poor Benjamin! O my dear innocent, my sweet prince! How I should love and pet you now if you were by my side and if I had not had the misfortune to become infatuated with a fine wit!' The coquette infused her invective with such a strong note of sincerity that I could not listen without being moved. How charming was my Manto's childlike and cunning anger! How gracious her sadness, whether real or feigned! To beg her pardon, to calm her grief, was an indescribable pleasure. I took her on my knee, I kissed and cradled her, I whispered tender words as one does with little girls; I drank her tears, I gently patted her cheeks, hot and bright as a beautiful precocious fruit, and said to myself: 'Imbecilic fop! Fabricator of illusions! Such sincerity, but also such baseness!'

"Not for anything in the world would I describe to you in detail those shocking scenes in which very rarely were tears the only things to flow. Besides, you seem to me in something of a hurry to be done with this Benjamin whom you don't know and for whom no doubt you care nothing. I have digressed at great length about him, but what can I do, chevalier? The misdeed has been committed. Am I not a man of digressions? And what does it matter? At any rate, before I return to my story, permit me to mention another of my rivals and friends: Milord Edward Gordon Colham, a young man who had recently arrived in Venice to learn about life and to waste his time as an embassy secretary. The amiable islander's youth and the expression of frankness and innocence emanating from his entire person straightaway caused la Mérone to permit him certain intimacies of a nature scarcely designed to please me. I soon recognized, however, that there was nothing in the foolish stripling's assiduous attentions to offend me, and in the end I even developed a certain taste for the charming Edward. In no time at all la Sulmerre was calling him little brother; I called him sweet. Milord played the spinet agreeably, had the most beautiful eyes and hair in the world, and seemed to find pleasure only in the company of effeminate men. I will spare you other details about him; at the outset, the role he played in the ludicrous drama of my love affair amounted to almost nothing, and in the remainder of my story we will see him reappear only once. Still, I consider it useful to tell you of the confidences which, in keeping with my deplorable habit, I lost no time in pouring out to him. Better than anyone else in the world you know already both the horrible anxiety which racked my mind and the atrocious love which devoured my heart.

"Life is holy and man is evil, and life takes revenge on man. From the first look I seemed to recognize in Clarice-Annalena the mysterious projection of the dear image so cherished long ago when I was a child; far from diminishing with time and habit, this delicious first impression only gained force and sharpness. To love la Mérone soon seemed to me a return to the lost sweetness of my early years. In the eyes of my beauty I rediscovered the sky and fountains of the duchy of Brettinoro; in her hair, the fragrance of the wind blowing from the familiar river and the fraternal forest; in her voice, the laughter and songs of the companions of my youth. I loved the sweet lady a little like an adolescent schoolboy and very much like a childishly incestuous little sister. Alas, Annalena! Alas! My childhood, my child, my childishness! There is nothing so agreeable in all the world, in my opinion, as the delight of discovering in a fallen woman some remnant of childish grace, of sweetness and purity. It is more fleeting than the melancholy of the last ray of the sun on the expanding cloud of night, and more delicate than the fragility of a flower picked at the season's end. Certainly the virgin in her innocence is lovable; but my nature is such that I shall prefer always to find a little when I least expect it to the joy of encountering a great deal when I am sure of finding it. A preference for the unforeseen has guided me in my loves as in all else, and to that I owe the pursuit of the dissolute life which I began in my youth, for no sooner would it become apparent that someone's feelings were feigned than I would feel the odd desire rise up in me to inspire real ones. Far from being defeated by the inevitable rebuffs that I suffered in this fantastic game, I amused myself by softening the effect of these rejections by interpreting them in a certain way. Against my strict, rational judgment I opposed all the arguments that seemed appropriate to encourage me to be indulgent; yet as nobility was necessary to me at any price, I opened my purse constantly and rejoiced naively when I found, failing love, a little gratitude in the heart of the venal women who comforted me.

"As thankless as was the task that I had set my heart on, nonetheless I found numerous occasions to compliment myself on my liberal and gallant optimism, especially in my relations with Annalena. The gratitude that she had become accustomed to show me on every occasion was not the only sentiment that astonished me in a woman of her age and condition. Although appreciative of the luxury with which I surrounded her, she appeared to value it less than the affectionate and honest manner in which I treated her in the presence of others. She brought to her most immodest transports a gentle tenderness which seemed to prove the sincerity of her feeling as much as the vivacity of her pleasure. The way she had also of forgiving faults was so charming that sometimes I suspected her of provoking deliberately my jealous rages. Her sulks were childish and touching, and there was an ingenuous grace even in her sins, for she was perverse in the manner of novices and nuns. Her little tears tasted of fairy rain from the blond kingdom of autumn of Riquet à la Houppe,* and how delicious I found it to kiss away her little grimaces of anger or disdain. Her bodice swelled at the slightest emotion, showing a bosom replete with all the charms of that delicate and troubling age when beauties cease to be young girls without being able to decide whether to become women entirely. Her body was like May rosebushes whose hard and trembling foliage offers to enchanted lips a small, stiff flower, barely open, smooth and bittersweet to kiss. But above all it was her laughter, Annalena's laugh! A laugh that was bright, rustic, primitive, fraternal; a child's laughter trembling with the murmurs of springs awakened in bygone days during a nocturnal halt in the midst of a strange forest; and deafened by the birdsongs of May heard in a half-sleep, in the depths of a misty orchard; and shivering from the sound of rain and hail on the roofs of the ancient chateau of Brettinoro; and somnolent from the songs of the wind in the desolate chimneys; and still moved by the sound of Christmases past. . . .

"That is what I believed I heard, I who never had encountered Love; yes, that is what I heard, I the most solitary, in the unique laugh of la Mérone, in that soft laugh which blossomed suddenly in my beauty's voice like a rose blazing on the rosebush, like the strange hail of autumn's gilded acorns falling from the rustling oak tree. And I closed my eyes, I hid my face . . . thirty years of uneasy solitude, of passionate expectation, of timid and nostalgic debauchery . . . thirty years of the soul's drought, the imagination's madness, the heart's impotence! When I was sixteen I read *Don Quixote de la Mancha* under the weeping willow of my ancestral park, and I waited, I waited near the murmuring fountain. Days followed days, seasons and years succeeded each other. . . . And I saw myself, in my dark dream, wandering the world aimlessly, wasting life, prodigal with gold and with the hours of youth; admired, flattered, celebrated everywhere, and for all that more miserable, in my heart's solitude, than the old beggar squatting at the entrance to the cemetery.

"Bizarre recollections of countries and of cities passed before my inner eye; landscapes of mist and sun, of winter and summer, of the South and the North; streets and lanes at evening and morning, silent or noisy; crowds of all countries and all races; the hospitality of palaces and cottages; docks, post houses, halts by rivers and daydreams of inns. . . . Ah, the feeling of melancholy and lassitude of arrivals mixed with the emptiness and regret of departures! And this overwhelming, atrocious certainty that the soul will be tomorrow what it is today, and what it was yesterday, and ten years ago, and all through eternity. . . .

"And then it was that a strange laugh resounded suddenly so far away, so far and so close to me! The laugh of an adolescent dear to my adolescence, a laugh from the past and of the future, a flowing and flowering laugh of a wild thing gentle as a soothing balm. . . . With eyes closed, my life hanging on this melody of youth, I was carried back, monsieur le chevalier, to my gloomy past of a rock lost amid the solitude of the seas; to my depressing past of the indifferent inn lamp, to my horrible past as an old canal measuring the days, years, and centuries of the monotonous flow of rust-poisoned rains. And when I opened my eyes again, I found before me my first love as a child, as an adolescent, and as a graybeard: Clarice-Annalena Mérone the adventuress! Clarice-Annalena Mérone, de Sulmerre, the hussy, alas!

"The bewitching strumpet had a strongly marked taste for childish gambols in front of mirrors, for which I often reproved her with a learned, severe air, for these solitary frolics caused me some jealousy; nonetheless, the contrite laugh of a schoolgirl caught in the wrong disarmed me in the twinkling of an eye, and the image of the tender Daphnis joined the reflection of the lovable Chloe. The accent which she adopted for her complaints and reprimands left me ravished with pleasure; her pronunciation was like that of a child, and when she said 'Savage!' I heard 'Sabbath'; 'vile!' I repeated 'wile'; 'tyrant!' I exclaimed 'tylant, tylant!'—and the minx burst out laughing, jumping for joy and clapping her hands. She invented games involving a patient and a doctor, a mischievous little girl and a strict mentor, a young beauty caught by surprise in a woodland by a brazen old man; and there followed delicious operations, exquisite flagellations, savage, anxious, intoxicating violations. She dressed as a young boy, and put on a belt whose buckle completed her body; and Enobarbus*-Pinamonte bounced Sporus*-Annalena on his knee. At other times she pretended to be a governess with a vituperative temper and wanted me to call her my beloved. Then she ordered me about, made me spell out from a large book, commanded me to recite my prayer or declaim some fable. Woe to the scatterbrained schoolboy! He quaked in his boots, I swear it! The whip was always within reach of the shrew. 'Two pigeons loved each other with a love . . .' 'So, monsieur, is that all you have learned? With a love . . ., go on, what are you waiting for, you wicked imp?' 'With a love . . ., madam, with a love that was ten-tender . . .' The small hand raised the large whip, and at the same time an undergarment was dropped, and there was this great beanpole of a Brettinoro on his knees in front of his beloved. 'Ah, the little libertine! What do I see? What does this mean? But it's a little man! What am I saying, a proficient bad boy? What rascal teaches you these fine things, you naughty man? I want to know at once, or else I'll have a word with Monsignor about it . . . Come now, don't cry, it's all right; get up and come here so that I can kiss you . . .' And my sweet love kissed me tenderly . . . 'With a love that is singular, childish, perverse, profound, and melancholy; a love most rare, my adored one! Come here so that I may give you back the same!' Ah! chevalier, how sweetly flowed the hours at the palazzo Mérone!

"Before meeting la Sulmerre I had never know any affection other than that which still today causes me to cherish the past to the point where my real existence is located there, and I seek no society other than old books and ancient objects. The phantom of regret binds us to life no less than the mirage of hope. By falling in love with la Mérone I drew her into the magic circle forbidden to my contemporaries; I dressed her as the heroine of a dusty novel; I gave her for company Agnes,★ Beatrix,★ and Laurette de Sado,★ and brought to her sweet old-fashioned child's face my rejuvenated soul, in which she might contemplate herself as in a beautiful old mirror bathed in the tears of love. All the madness of my senses and all the wisdom of my soul was contained in my affection. My mind dwelt ceaselessly on my Mérone; my life was nourished by the dear life of the enchantress. In pronouncing the names of the ravishing one I discovered in my voice the mysterious inflection of sacred words, and I whispered 'Clarice' as one murmurs 'Queen of the angels'; I said 'Annalena' as one sighs 'pray for us.' My lungs recognized the air breathed by the beloved, my eyes gathered from flowers the dear gaze that had rested on them; objects gave back to my hands caresses received from the fingers of the adored one, and sweet nature in its entirety presented itself to me with the magnificent features of a great Annalena, omnipotent and eternal. Love permitted me to penetrate the essence of my being; a new kind of Pythagoras, I discovered in myself a world governed by mystical numbers. Annalena was the sure and inconceivable unity from which were derived in endless combinations the affections of my soul and the associations of my thoughts. Love is an attraction, and infinite gravitation is itself

---

merely a perceptible form of universal love. The image of my dearest was more faithful than my shadow, for the body's shadow mingles with the shadows and dissolves in them, whereas the beloved ghost followed me through the night into the fearful depths of dreams.

"One time, only once, did I succeed in escaping my delicious obsession in sleep. This act of rebellion, even though unconscious, brought a terrible punishment upon me. From this dream without Annalena I woke stupefied and filled with anguish, in the midst of darkness. La Sulmerre was far from my thoughts; my dream had taken me back to the time of my first youth, and I thought that I was in my narrow bed in the old chateau of Brettinoro. Suddenly, as I move, I become aware that there is a strange body next to mine. The image of Annalena immediately regains its place in my mind, and yet a horrible feeling of distress grips my heart. I listen . . . not a breath . . . I cry out: 'Annalena! Annalena! My dear love!' No reply; nothing moves. Finally, I pick up the lighter; the spark shoots up, the candle is lit; and here is Annalena pale as a toppled statue whitened by the moon, so close to me, so close and yet so far, so far! Wandering in the country of dreams, entwined in the high grasses of silence, a stranger, lost, almost dead . . . Terrible, how terrible is the face of sleep! So close to me, and in the depths of what abyss, in the heart of what mystery! There you are, then, you! O you, you who are everything! You next to me, who is so alone! Poor you, poor us! The night. The silence. This pale restless torch, this old palace inhabited by strange memories . . . on the wall, the enormous, frightening, baroque shadow of this great beanpole in a nightshirt . . . Who is she?

From whence does she come? Who am I? Where am I going? She did not live in my dream of a moment ago and doubtless I do not exist in hers. What abyss separates us! What are we doing here? I spread a handkerchief on her face, and her name is forgotten, lost, erased; her body has no name; decapitated, even she would not recognize it. What a life! What an eternity! What stench of the charnel-house! She lived for a long time knowing nothing of me, alas, nothing, not even the name. And she slept alone or in the arms of another, in this same position! And I went gallivanting far off! The cold, the shadow on the sea, the unknown, silence everywhere! Yes, the moonlight on white Russia and on the steeples black with crows. . . . And the moonlight on the chateau of the Grand Duke of Mazovie and on Windsor!—Tomorrow is approaching. Tomorrow can bring only pain. Tomorrow is always a separation. Eternity itself is only the time of a goodbye, a leaf's fall, the flash of a tear.—I shout at the top of my voice: 'Horror! Horror!—Heaven, what a laugh! How she laughs, this imp of an Annalena!'—'I have been watching you for some time, my very dear monsieur; tell me, Sassolo, have you lost your mind? What are you doing? Why are you not asleep? Blow out the candle, please. I am dying of sleep. Kiss me hard, calm yourself, good night.'—Peace returns to my soul. I blow; a fly burns its wing . . . I blow; it hits against the ceiling. Silence. I blow again. Now there is the night, and the rain. Such tranquility, such sweetness. All is in order again. In what order, O my peculiar mind? In the order of things, apparently. Ah! . . . Bah! The great beanpole yawns. Shadows. The sound of rain on the canal. La Mérone's hair smells of spring hay in the moonlight. . . . And there, monsieur le chevalier, there you have our friend Pinamonte, my friend Myself, peacefully falling asleep again—like a May ass drunk with young hay.

"A short time after our first meeting in the palace of B——, I had to go to Milan about a matter of succession. A slight indisposition prevented la Mérone from joining me. I had been there about two or three days when one evening, crossing the Via Paolo da Cannobio, near the cathedral, I was struck by the sorry state of a house which appeared to be the doyen of this street so full of memories. It is drizzling softly. The plaintive sounds of a harpsichord can be heard in the distance. Here you have our friend Pinamonte in the midst of a dream; it seems to him that the door, above which is the coat of arms of the Ricci family, invites him; the threshold is crossed, the long corridor traversed, and then there is a small colonnaded courtyard whose paving stones are broken, loose, and covered with moss. In a dark corner, the leprous head of a chimera spits a small stream of greenish water into a muddy basin. Pinamonte lifts his nose and stares wide-eyed. 'It is the house of the Past, it is the house of the Past,' croons this devil of a harpsichord. 'Look carefully, friend Pinamonte; are not these murky high windows to your taste? Annalena lived there a hundred years ago. She watered the flowers in the window on the left every morning, every morning a hundred years ago. In the old days, the poor old days long gone.'—A window opens, the hideous head of an old woman wearing a monstrous bonnet calls to me: 'It's this way, there, the little door on your left; enter, enter, please . . . There are three steps . . . You are M. Spallantini, isn't that so? The dancing master? Come, come; M. de Tassistro has been waiting for you for several hours.' Instead of answering I remain fixed there, confused. I blush, I cough, I blow my nose, I raise my hand to my hat. What should I do, by the Styx! What excuse can I give, by the Devil! Won't the old harridan take me for a thief, an assassin? I stammer the devil knows what: 'Old house, my good woman; love of the past, curiosity . . . a stranger passing through Milan, slightly drunk, problems. . . .' Then I take flight, and in one bound reach the middle of the street.

"Months after this memorable event I find myself in Annalena's boudoir. It is summer. It is hot. I am idle. I am bored. I pick up a book, leaf through it distractedly, throw it down. I watch the flight of a fly. It alights on the window, and there is the great silence of a June evening. Ah! I spy a little jewel box. I pick it up, open it, and, while daydreaming mindlessly, toss the jewelry in my hand. I reflect vaguely upon my last voyage; in my thoughts I see again my dear cathedral, the Via Cannobio, the house of the Past. My hand keeps bouncing. A ring falls. I pick it up and examine it minutely, all the while musing about other things. I notice a date incised in the ring. I go over to the window: '1708. P. Tassistro.' I cross myself, I swear, I call Clarice, I question her. She had not ever noticed the inscription. The ring had come to her from a great-aunt. Never had she heard of the Tassistro family. There is a great mystery at the bottom of every affection, an impenetrable secret in the heart of every passion; a dream that one forgets upon waking, a silence that one dares not trouble, a word one is afraid to say.

"I have loved intensely; I have the right to speak. But woe to him who takes the name of the Eternal in vain! Nothing is more foreign to our pitiful comprehension than this terrible sweet love which is the principle of human beings, and which causes our heart to commingle with a pebble in the road, for we have trouble enduring life and our love is intoxicated with eternity. All that may have existed before us is hidden, all that must out-live us a mystery; nevertheless, the mind is loath to separate the idea of love as much from what we were before making our appearance in this world as from what we shall be after leaving it, and the fact of being able, during our temporal sojourn, to love dissimilar beings at different times with the same love is perhaps the strongest argument against those who deny immor-tality. Loves pass and die; love remains and survives, and such is the power of the earthly forms in which it manifests itself—art, enthusiasm, beauty—that it always finishes by prevailing over falsehood, father of ugliness and madness. Love is that which remains and which constitutes the personality. If we open the incoherent book of our past we are much surprised to read the story not of the individual whom we thought we were, but of a turbulent crowd of strangers. And if we have the pleasure of meeting someone there who bears a slight resemblance to what we are today, let us be very careful not to speak to him of any-thing other than sentiment!

"My primary care with la Mérone was always to conceal my thoughts from her. The sweet thing came from too far away; she was my dear sentimental ghost of the wild gardens of Brettinoro; she was the hidden sense of my life, the shape of my existence outside of time; of the words that I spoke to her, none related to anything of the present; and the amorous sim-plicity of my remarks continuously astonished me. How primitive am I! I said to myself; what does this mean, what is the significance of that? Am I then an inhabitant of Saana?* How nature sings in my voice! Dead forests shuddering, strange extinct birds beating their wings, childish prayers to the sun, to the moon, to the silence, to the wind! The feeling that all this already has been said long ago, a very long time ago, before, before, always before, much before everything! Here is the word, the numerous word with but one meaning, the tender, mysterious translucent language of seasons renewed, of worlds destroyed and reborn, passing sounds in the canticle with no beginning or end! And I repeated, 'My dear life, my great thrilling angel, my deeply beloved! Your eyes, your hands, your knees, your mouth! Your footprints in the dust, your voice in the night, your sleep underneath the moon, your hair in the wind! Why are you like a flower on the water, like a nest in the crook of a tree, and like the echo in the menacing forest?' I spoke these poor and holy things, and in each word I found the word of the enigma of the world. . . .

"At times, while contemplating the sky and the sea, I felt so powerful an emotion rise from the depths of my soul that the most sublime sight was diminished by it; and all I could find to bear witness to my love were the blandishments of an old man weeping over a cradle. 'Here is the life-giving ocean, created, explored, and enclosed in the night,' I cried to myself, 'and here is the night, measured and enveloped by light! The plaintive wind has risen; my amorous thoughts go beyond the wind, farther than Venus scintillating up there. How small the ring of realities seems to those who embrace it from the spiritual center! Yes, but it is truly small, small and charming enough to make one laugh, this childish universe offered to my terrible affection! I barely understand it and I acknowledge it; the most pathetic thing is beyond my comprehension: a grain of sand in the road, a tear from the sea, the motion of a gull's wings. But what does it matter if my mind will never completely understand this loving eternity delivered to my love? Does not drawing closer to things, dissolving in them, result only in knowing oneself a stranger to one's own understanding? I do not know the reasons of life but I sense them, and I sense that love and beauty can do anything, anything except 'not to be.' Tender, tender things! Tender and profound! How much you need my pity in order to survive! How your infiniteness would frighten you if the idea of the infinite was not my love itself! What harmony reigns between us! Am I not in you, are you not in me? Such sweetness in us and outside of us, such wisdom both necessary and irrational! And how well made is this great moving orb for understanding the movement of my immense heart! Love, beginning and end, Love and love. Here you are, I cried wildly, here you are at last, O Love! How sweet is your presence! and how terrible is your shadow alongside mine! Before we met you were only a God to me, a poor personal God; a God in heaven and a fear in the heart of man; and here you are yourself finally, and you are love, love and pain! Yes, pain, O, certainly! pain; for you have stripped yourself of your mystery. You passed all understanding in the old days of your divinity; you were unimaginable; your name was Infinite; the date of your arrival was Future.

"And now you are there, close to me, you the incessant creation, you the thing that has no need to know itself, you the newborn's first cry! O Love, the infinite divested of mystery, God in his sublime nakedness, overwhelming necessity, ruler of Reason, Christ in the world of bread and wine and birth. You, perfect language after the infantile stammering of sages; you, the eternal idea or the undiscoverable thing for one, the obvious will for the other; you who can be neither idea nor thing nor will, being yourself! O terrible Presence! O Infinite divested of mystery! what poetry, what music, what painting, what dance will ever express the eternity of your own astonishment before the splendor of being yourself! Come! Embrace me! Let us go toward the gardens that are on the seas! Let us go toward the springs that are in the forests! Let us trample with our human step the sand which caresses, and the stone which rends, and the dust of the moon which makes everything old! And let us proclaim, so that our children will hear, the gods of all ages and of all races! And may I be no longer man and may you be no longer woman; for you are love in me, and we are the supreme unity formed of two earthly unities! And let us go awaken, under the oak tree dazzled by the wind, she who was our shared bed, Clarice-Annalena, pitiful and pale in the world of bread and wine and birth. Come, Love, embrace me! You whose feet are lower than any abjectness and whose head is more radiant than any light! Song of the constellations, small harmonious curve on the Phrygian shell, harp of the rising sun, refuge of the winds, foaming rapture of the seas! You who have made eternity known to me! Son of the living God! 'Your face shines like the sun, your clothes are white as light!'

"Like a sleepless man, I draw near to you, O window filled with sunlight and humming with flies, O Love, window open to life! And here I see the moment of the wave, and the wink of an eye gleaming with foam, and the flash of a white wing in the midst of the blindness of the waters! Space, space that separates the waters; my joyous friend, how I breathe you in with love! Here I am like a nettle flowering in the gentle sunlight of ruins, and like a pebble on the rim of the spring, and like a snake in the heat of the grass! What, is the moment truly eternity? Is eternity truly the moment? Vanity of human dreams, blacknesses of pride and dishonesty, I mock you in the soft laugh of drunken flies! Shivering little palm tree offered to the steel wind, little stone shining in the laughing foam, and you, unhappy man in rags, chewing your miserable bread in the presence of the fearsome splendors of the Son of Man! What wisdom there is in you! How I love you! How sweet it is to me to be the most secret heartbeat of immortal flesh! O eternity! What a gentle master, what an amorous brother you have found in me! With what generosity I exalt you with all the haste of my human moments! With what certainty I predict your future, great sentimentalist who still does not yet know itself! For fierce love will come back, awful truth is very near. And I know under which wave the stone shines, the stone which must shatter the mouth of falsehood, ugliness, and madness! For soon they will tear themselves apart, the old smothering horizons, finally revealing the distances of music and the honey of consolation! Who would deny it, when all of my flesh burns with prophecies! Who would mock it, when all of the final revelation already is passionately kissing my blood with its blazing lips? Secret lust of being, throbbing in the belly of life, swelling of tenderness in the heart of hearts, I feel you, you penetrate me with all your fury, your humid hotness is on my mouth, your tears lacerate my face.

"Ah, imperfect old world of joyful news! How you teeter on the edge of eternity! Come to my heart, O accomplished world, O common cradle and grave of an unclean race! I love you with all the despair of last moments! Already your bleached sky trembles like a rag stained with the tears of farewell! Ah, how I love you, ancient vestige of a dying world, old skin of a sickly beast! O Love! do not harm it! Do not avenge yourself too well! Let it die its death! Pardon this world where you had no kingdom, forget the spittle on the face and the nails in the bones, and let it be, let it be (for everything was so well thought out! All that was missing was one more drop of bitterness, only one, only one, for everything to have been achieved!) Forget, o my lover! Do not smite it; let it rot quietly in its sleep. See, its poor teeth are broken already! The stone is in the throat; the old viper can find no exit. And what does it matter to you? Are you not luxuriously reclining on the heart's throne? Do you not have my eyes on yours? Do I not stand before you, eternity before eternity, love before Love! Let it rot quietly!

"You laugh, my lover! Serpent, you say? Ah, you are only sun and laughter! But understand, my beloved, there is good in the serpent's caution! Powerful, powerful! Also surprising, and delectable! And profound, yes, profound! More profound than the heavens and the seas and the lands of which you are the principle and the essence! More profound than all the ancient desires of God! Profound, profound, profound! *Raison d'être,* heart, amorous evidence of all things! You who turn the awesome infinite into a sweet little thing to hold in your hand; you who are part of all matter until now considered unconscious; you who enter into all of radiant nature; you through whom bread and wine become his flesh and his blood, and for whom his death is the dimming of the sun; O Consoler, to whom we lift our blind eyes! I have heard you singing in the night with the voice of the sea, on anguished sands! Many a time have I seen your shadow bend over Magdalen's slumber! I have felt you tremble in the poorest and most lifeless things. Stone of solitary and sinister shores, you have beat against my heart! O rose, what wisdom you exhale! What learning comes from you, insensate insects, in the dark honeyed light of evening! Snows of the peaks, rags of the poor, mists over the *faubourgs,* with what fervor one and the same principle pervades you! O God in my flesh! O God in my tenderness, O God whom I touch, observe! How beautiful is the beloved!

"And you, you whose heartbeat measures infinity, how humble and near you are, Love! Thing in itself, reason infinitely necessary to all things, God dispersed and unique, master of Will, commander of Reason, unfathomable to Science, road made of Feeling! You are on me, under and above me, and you are in me! Ah, sweet word that has never been uttered! Ah, devastating certitude of simplicity! How you envelop me, how you caress me, how you insinuate yourself in the flesh of my heart! Truly, wasn't it only that? So many labors, so many quests and combats and separations! That and only that? The subtle, profound, insupportable certainty of Love! O most ingenuous of revelations! But what tomorrow! What vengeance! What ghastly vengeance! What crumbling of the rottenness of pride and of falsehood! What plague upon men and upon the heavens! Then what beauty, what calm, what horizon of love unveiled for all eternity!

"O future of perfect love, alone before yourself, how near you are! New man! How the sound of your step multiplies! Fall, boundaries with no love of horizons! Appear, true distances! One: revelation. Two: waiting. Three: approach. Four: awful turbulence. Five: stone of the Truth that smashes teeth. Six: deliverance. Seven: ecstasy, ecstasy! Eternity of ecstasy!

"Sometimes the tumult of my feelings was so great, the movement of my heart so precipitate, the desire to pour forth my soul in a single cry so impetuous that, deeming vain and contaminated by reason not only the words on my lips but also the most ardent evocations of sacred texts, I renounced the pleasure of even borrowing from the language of men an expression for the overflow of my emotion and of my gratitude. Then, as if blown by the wind of madness, I hurried to the street; I pressed to my heart men, women, and children; I tossed in the air handfuls of money and jewels, laughing until the tears came if I happened to overhear the influence of wine blamed for what I knew to be a result of the sagest emotion. 'They always have the poor,' and 'Him, Him, they no longer have.' Avidly I kissed the sunstruck stones, the trees mute with the heat, the lazy, odorous water of the canals; without making any distinction, I wrapped all of nature in my love, the slightest things with the most important, the repulsive as well as the attractive; blind and deaf matter seemed to me to be impregnated with love down to the most infectious germs, just as the worst of men has in him something of the angel.

"Admittedly, with the passage of time my cruel reason has

not ceased to find something of the ridiculous in the memory of those touching, ardent days; nevertheless, the exaltation I felt then seems to me even today much more excessive in its expression than unreasonable in its essence. Am I not, in effect, indebted solely to love for all this belated knowledge vainly pursued in the scribblings of men? Did it not teach me to seek the salt of the earth in the places where there was still some chance of discovering it? Did it not tell me, finally, to give myself over to life as the sleeper abandons himself to dreams and to transpose into reasoned reality all the sweetness of the affective world of dreams? Ah, chevalier, it is this last influence especially which made me value the wisdom of love above all others! For dreams have the salutary power to make us burn with a greater flame for that which is beautiful, to shake us with a more violent revulsion at the spectacle of vile things and to elicit from us more burning tears at the sight of adversity. If things appear larger to us in dreams, more beautiful, more touching, or more horrible, it is because they are measured by the power of feeling freed from the bonds of reason. The simple fact that certain dreams reproduce with more or less fidelity images received by the senses suffices sometimes to engender profound doubts; what are these doubts, however, compared to the confidence we gain in reconciling that which governed us when awake and that which guides us in dreams? Emotion offers us the deep mirror of dreams, and how surprised we are to recognize ourselves in the features of universal love! Thanks to this divine game, we learn that the exterior world is real only insofar as the intelligence which animates it is the reflection of emotion burning in the core of being, for everything outside of us comes from that which is inside us. In the same way that the soul is the expression of the love of God for God himself, the object is the form of the love of man for man. All the same, even though infinite Love which, embracing all things, necessarily contains the notion of the imperfect and therefore burns with an adoration of itself ever more passionate, we exist as an object for the sole design of magnifying, by the continual creation of beauty, this unique certitude, this supreme reality of an interior world that is all love.

"If we cherish temporal existence, it is not at all because we come from it, but for the reason that in finding in it what is necessary to realize the beauty that is epitomized by our soul, we glorify both the creature among creatures whom we are and that original love whose need to adore itself more and more presents itself to us in our conception of the infinite. For the thing without end never could be that in itself, but only as an attribute of love; and it is in its nature, like desire in the finite being, to be a movement unlimited by that even though it can have no purpose outside of itself. As for our idea of nothingness, I perceive its origin in an imagination distorted by Mendacity, that arrogant and sterile contradictor, that impotent enemy of amorous evidence. In the eyes of the mystic, the world is all affirmation; could it be otherwise in the perceptible manifestation of a God whose power has no other limit than the impossibility of not being love, that is to say, of not being? True life is an initiation by feeling. If we have called love by the supreme name of Creator from the earliest times it is because neither the mind nor the senses sufficed to make our temporal sojourn a reality. For true life is not that which comes to us, but rather that which comes from us. To be is to create, not to receive, one's life; and love is the unique instrument of an infinity of possible creations. That which we call reality is not something which offers itself to us, but a fruit of initiation, and initiation commences with love. Thus it is not only ingenious, logical, or sublime, but absolutely necessary to identify, in the terrestrial sense, the science of the Divine with a Beatrice born from one flesh and one soul. Heaven is not a feverish dream: the roads that lead to it are made of sand and rock permeated with love, so gorged with love as to make one weep; thus, before undertaking the conquest of so formidable a reality, let us try to fill ourselves with real love during our preparatory life in time.

"No doubt the secrets of my past which I am confiding to you already strike you as too strange for me to be permitted to add a detailed description of visions more fantastic yet. Therefore I will restrict myself to relating only one of those countless dreams in which my too-human love presented itself to me with its retinue of emotions, doubts, terrors, and disgusts. I was subject to onsets of drowsiness that overtook me during the day, often at the height of an animated discussion, and sometimes even in the noisiest street. A feeling of dryness in the throat, a prickling around the eyes, and a great hollowness in my entire body usually preceded the attack. I then had just enough time to drag myself to my bed, and no sooner did I sink onto it than I fell into a heavy sleep like a desperate man jumping into a well with a stone around his neck. I remained in an unconscious state for an hour or two, after which I awoke as suddenly as I had fallen asleep, sometimes bursting out in peals of laughter, sometimes crying hot tears. Now, this is what happened to me

during one of these strange naps: I found myself in a most aris-
tocratic palace, whose style and furnishings greatly intrigued me
by the way in which they were so much in accord, by the sureness of taste, and by an indefinable originality. My head high,
one hand on my sword and the other on my hip, my hat under
my arm, nobly balancing myself on tiptoe, emaciated and full
of arrogance, I went through rooms and galleries on the arm of
an old gentleman who showed me around the house. Despite
the nice manners of my host, his good-natured smile and amusing
remarks, I was not particularly pleased by the conversation; and
each time that my eyes met those of the old man I felt a disquiet all the more disturbing because I sought to no avail in his
honest face some sign that would justify it. I had no knowledge
whatsoever of the place where I found myself nor of the purpose that had brought me there; still less did I recall ever having
met the jovial person who made me so welcome and whom
with hypocritical familiarity I called 'My dear marquis de
Lamorthe.' As we strolled through an interminable series of sitting rooms, the master of the house told me curious little stories
of his life at court as well as smutty anecdotes of inns and camps,
but I did not allow myself to be distracted from my gloomy
reverie by the magnificence of what met my gaze nor by the
somewhat offensive raciness. I was oppressed by the bizarre feeling that something dreadful, a creature with no name, an unknown monster, was watching me from some hiding place and
waited only for a signal from this dear marquis to make itself
visible to me in all its horror. Every fiber of my body was tense
with waiting: in dreams, time is so deep, so heavy, so hostile!
Finally we stopped in front of a large window that opened onto

a park that I judged, or rather guessed, to be immense; for the high wall surrounding it rose up very close to the window and hid all but the upper branches of motionless old trees, dark and thick. The marquis ceased his banter and began to observe me furtively. A supernatural silence deprived of all movement, not just the simple absence of voices; an almost repulsive melancholy drenching everything in a lifeless light; the absurd proximity of the wall built there as if for the sole purpose of concealing from view a garden which was undoubtedly very beautiful. . . . My anguish became intolerable. I was suffocating in that silent hell. I needed at all costs to hear a sound even if it was only my own voice. In my distress I murmured, 'Heavenly powers! How strange this is!' The marquis then smiled sweetly at me, winked his eye, nodded his head, and the following colloquium ensued before that ghastly wall: *The marquis:* Well, of course life is a remarkable thing. Ah, the philosophers! Let us cultivate our garden! And here is the only garden that one cultivates reasonably . . . the only one, by my faith, there, before our eyes. And the old humdrum routine continues in spite of everything. The same sky, the same sun; the same love, too, especially the same love. Don't you find the smell of this garden quite delicious? *I:* Certainly, but that wall. . . . *The marquis:* Ah, that wall. Ah, yes, that wall. Nevertheless . . . to the devil with the wall! What does it matter to me? I have air here and I don't care about the rest. *I:* But it seems to me that the view would be more attractive . . . couldn't you have it knocked down? *The marquis:* Yes, I agree that the trees there are quite beautiful, and if it were only up to me . . . but this is not my property. *I:* Is that possible? But then, who is the fortunate . . . *The marquis:* The neighboring village,

Vercelli. And the whole province. Moreover, they are thinking about enlarging it. It's already quite congested. *I:* I understand: Sundays, no doubt? The riffraff of the neighborhood? *The marquis:* Yes, but a considerable number of persons of quality as well. Thanks to that . . . to that (give me the word, monseigneur) that notorious dissolute woman . . . *I:* Really! A creature? And who then? *The marquis:* No, you could not imagine anything more farcical! Really! Hundreds—What am I saying! Thousands. . . . *I:* But is this Cythera,* here? Ah, my dear marquis, I suspect you of . . . *The marquis:* Yes; thousands, caravans, legions. Legions of admirers! And with all the trappings! Real baboons, my dear count-duke. Sometimes also tears, sighs, moaning, crowns, torches. . . . They come from all corners of the world. Officers, members of the legal profession, men of letters, even churchmen. What a world! Really! A singular mélange of the obscene and the macabre! Lust and putrefaction. Flowers and vermin. Love, romance in a cemetery! And all for one Annalena de Mérone, a dead prostitute, a rottenness of rot! Truly, the decay of morals. . . .' The dear marquis did not have time to finish. A cry—and then the awakening. Horrible, horrible awakening! Since that night, chevalier, the simple sight of a cemetery wall fills me with fear and disgust.

"Emotion is the only reality. All the rest is but a mirage in temporal life as in dreams. Thus, in reopening my eyes to the light of hours so full of love, I had the twofold feeling of coming out of a dream and of returning to a dream. I know from experience the brutal or caressing action of all stimulants, all narcotics; many times have I crossed the plain ablaze with poppies, and in my barque woven of Indian hemp I have measured the interstellar vastnesses. Miserable inventions! Vile counterfeits! Nothing equals the bittersweet grass full of summer, silence, and storm, of hair which knots itself around our sadness like pliant seaweed around a drowned body! Nothing equals the pulsating fruit of an inexhaustible mouth where our memories sing, our desires moan, and our regrets lament! Nothing equals the fascinating and dreaded look which comes from farther away than life, which goes beyond death; nothing equals the quivering flesh that rises up, flower of Saana,* great thunderous aloe, toward the mystical magnet of the sun, the sun, direct satellite of love! Mysterious and sacred flesh! Vessel of feeling! Visible sign of prayer! Radiant blossoming of certitude! Holy clay, still swooning from the caress of the divine workman! O swift form of universal feeling! Here are kisses full of time and bitterness, sad and beautiful as the measured gaze of the stars; and here is formidable Maternity, and pale Sterility, sublime also in her prostitute's pain, and holy, holy, holy! like birth itself. And here, finally, on the heaving altar, the marriage of imperious soul and faithful flesh, of omnipotent feeling and obedient reason!

"All that, chevalier, all that have I known, seen, touched. Oh yes, my love was terrestrial, impure; wild, diseased, bitter wheat ravaged by the blight of disgust and senility . . . What does it matter! The worm attacks the purest things. When Adoration is there, profound and burning, is not the worst aberration a mere peccadillo? Alas, I remember. The sea whispered on the sands of the Lido; an uncommonly beautiful shadow clasped my shadow; all was light, sweetness, and wisdom; and in the unreal air distance signaled to distance. My love enclosed the universe; all the eternity of happiness moaned in my throat;

and my former anguish was reduced to a faint stain of shadow on the shining rock. 'What then do you continue to search for, God's blood, O Pinamonte, you insatiable imbecile! Is not everything closer to you than you yourself? Do you not hear rising from your heart the seething of the source of worlds? Does not your love suffice then? Is not the thing that consumes itself fire? The being who loves, is he not Love? Son of man, the key is in your hands. Only the blind man curses the useless key, but you, you who have eyes—what am I saying!—you who have eyes and SEE!' Alas, no! something was still missing. The sob of new joy choked me. 'I am thirsty! I am still thirsty! All bitterness has not been drunk; there is surely enough left to fill a sponge!'* With my arms crossed I stretched out on the shore. And the Sun nailed me to the earth!

"After these frenzies of the heart, these turmoils of the spirit, there were long hours not of calming down, not of resignation, but more like absolute indifference toward worldly things, more like perfect forgetfulness of self. Then a boundless shadow fell on my brain, shades of before and after the Sun, and I became again an infinity of immobile matter, formless and rough, where everything is already contained and nothing more reveals itself. I contemplated my shape as if it were something absurdly far away and subject to my will. And suddenly, something sweet and profound and tender, the Word: something enormous and infinitesimal, unprecedented and eternal, breaking the patient monotony of my being, began to stir madly with hope, joy, terror, insatiability—to whirl madly with impatience, triumph, affirmation, certainty—to spin madly with an obscure, inexplicable, undefined, uncoercible force—terrible hunger for adoration and attestation—horrible cry of demented joy in the infinity of the night; sublime devouring light in the sightlessness of the Abyss. O first revelation! I burn, I whirl, I explode; I am impatience, I am hunger, I am thirst! What a trail of flame behind me! How I run, how I fly to where the mad sand of the suns calls me! Who among them will be mine, will be the lover, the master, the guide? And what does it matter! They are without number, they are infinite Reality, consequently none of them is real! I am drunk, I cry out with desire, I am dying of love, I die of love eternally! How enchanted I am by the melody of my ellipsis! How profound is the moment! How it contains all that is, all that has been, all that will be! How rich I am in God! Love has made me fertile; my belly of sun vibrates with joy. Have I been this diaphanous disorderly form? Have I been it really? Bah! . . . For I am sun and sensibly installed for a new instant of eternity. And here I am Earth, great stone extinguished and maternal, lover of the sun, torn, furrowed, plowed, convulsed with the torment of love's juices. And like Love her master, full of joy and pain, of life and death, of remembrance and expectation. And then . . .

"And then an ordinary word, an ordinary mournful truth coming from a life whose reality is the first lie, a world which is not the kingdom of love; a syllable, a look, a smile, a gesture, anything at all dissipated in the blink of an eye all the treasures of illusion. 'A lovely spectacle,' I grumbled between my shaky old teeth, 'What a lovely spectacle of an idiotic ass wallowing at the feet of a predatory, silly strumpet! Empty old brainless skull, shell of a rotten nut, hole filled with night and with necrophagous insects, when will you cease to feed upon mirages? Madness, wake from your misfortune; old age, recognize your ugliness; cadaver, smell your stench. It really becomes you to play Adam before the lie! Recognize who you are, finally, look! There you are in an evil place where plague has penetrated, where the serpent of the tomb creeps into vulvas, where the wind of putrefaction breathes on funereal beds. O cursed house of loveless fornication! Here the bread of life is full of blight and vermin, and the wine of life smells of the morning after a drinking bout. Come on, get up, you handsome Don Juan with hollow ribs, take this torch, go over to the bed, pull the beautiful purple curtain, a shipwreck's sail inflated with a mute wind of destruction. . . . Ah, you tremble, you old coward! You know that what is lying there is only the corpse of your dream. The corpse of youth, the putrefaction of beauty, the ignoble ghost of what was truth and splendor on the first day. . . . Go on, lie down on top of your Clarice, on your stupid, shameless, rapacious one! Corpse, your place awaits you in that common ditch of lying fornications and lusts without love! Filth, go bury yourself in the hospital sewer; hyena, go lick the knees of your dear great liquefying cadaver!'

"Nothing can pass through your mind, now, my dear chevalier, that did not pass through mine then. However bewitched was my poor brain, nonetheless I had retained all of my usual lucidity for ordinary things. I brought to my worst extravagances a concern for order, proportion, and method which astonished me more each day. Sometimes the light of a supernatural wisdom illuminated my deplorable heart and penetrated the farthest reaches of my being. I no longer doubted my effective reality; I lived, the entire universe was condensed in me, I disseminated myself throughout the universe. I possessed love and love possessed me; my joy was a martyrdom, my grief an ecstasy. I reread all the books of the Truth. I relived the *Gospels,* I loved the *Imitation,* the *Divine Comedy,* I admired Pascal. I pardoned brother Jean-Jacques. Certain poverties of the *Vita Nuova* surprised me. I penetrated to the very heart of life. Poets, in singing of love, particularly enjoy celebrating its tonic effect on the heart and the imagination; as for me, I am more and more inclined to think that the supreme virtue of that sentiment extends to all of nature, from the matter which we consider inanimate to the essential glands of our brain. I believe that the exaltation caused by deep affection is as beneficial to the philosopher as to the saint or the poet; for my own experience taught me to consider love as a manner of universal correspondence between matter and mind, and as a conscious expression of their identity in the presence of the unique Being. Source of existence, it seemed to me to be at the same time the unquestionable principle and the unique and perfect sense. Lovely, terrible mystery, instigator of all true thought, art, and science, it appears to primordial intellects in the symbolic numbers and forms which it later reduces to the logical trinity of eternal Creation, Matter, and Spirit; then, crowning the slow process of initiation, it attains unity in the divine person of the Consoler and in that way appears to us in its clearest and most touching form.

"Yes, chevalier of my heart, Love, the bizarre divinity that Fable describes as blind, love and love alone made me apprehend the secret of things and the mystery of my own thoughts. Revealing itself to me in the form of a supreme logic of Sentiment, it made itself known as the foundation of our entire spiritual architectonics. Thanks to it I learned to look for nothing else in divergent methods but the elements of a character study, so much so that now the only value to my mind in sublime but irreconcilable systems lies in their quality of more or less faithful expressions of different sensibilities. The famous philosophical spirit begins with an often unconscious observation of Sentiment which is its source and ends with a mystical confession before the Universe of love; for it is impossible to imagine other conclusions to the unhappy task of a dialectic convinced at the outset of the futility of its efforts. A pathetic game indeed, the schemings of our understanding! Our mind, simultaneously impatient and painstaking, is perfectly aware of its powerlessness to go beyond the limits imposed by its own laws, yet it insists on investigating in depth, on continuously commenting upon the purely amorous acts of God; but this effort can only conclude in enunciating with a precision more discouraging each day the natural reasons for our incapacity. Taken as a whole, understanding, a secondary faculty, seems to have been given to man for the sole purpose of enlightening him concerning the cardinal importance of Sentiment, and of guiding him accordingly in his research into the very principle of Being. Before we undertake the great conquest of heaven, we must learn to consider our precious Reason not as an independent and precise quality but only as the complement of an interior force hidden and unassessed until now. Alas! we barely know yet how to love, and we would like to be able to reason!

"But especially because it has enlightened me as to the mystical meaning of the Word, I feel an ardent, limitless gratitude toward wise and tender Love. Because of it I know the secret significance of words, that indefinable something that is dormant in each word and changes according to the truth or falseness of the word. La Mérone, in this respect similar to all fallen women, was only too disposed to tricks; her conversation aroused my continual distrust; yet deep feeling interpreted in its own way the slightest sound of the adored voice. While my intelligence scented deceit or discovered lies, my soul abandoned itself without reserve to the indisputable miraculous truths of love; feeling accepted as truth that which reason rejected as false; human Mendacity spoke, but it was Love who listened, joyous, profound, triumphant Love! Ah, Mendacity! The vile contradictor! The trivial, cowardly enemy! Naive and ludicrous murderer, stupid profaner of the holinesses of love, it digs an insuperable chasm between reason and feeling, and thus appears to every thinking being as the source of the worst social calamities and the point of departure for the most fearsome diseases of the mind. To the ingenuous and proud gaze of Sentiment, all of sweet nature appears adorned with power, tenderness, and splendor; before Adam's lie, man knew no kingdom other than that of grace and harmony, and, heroic and confident, lived in the bosom of four primitive elements which are elements of pure beauty. Nature having retained order and splendor, a logical life should even today be profound adoration, for the thing called Beauty when it is outside of us is called Love when it is within us. Man's first idea was that of the love which he found in himself, in existence, in things. Fraternal confidant of animals, friend of stones, primitive man ruled over nature with the artlessness of Adam and the charm of Orpheus. Eating the fruit of life was not by any means his misfortune; it was renouncing, in the face of Love itself, sacred knowledge and holy delight. Drunk with pride and power, he found the first *no* when everything was *yes,* when everything around him was affirmation. And instead of hastening to the call of the Father, he hid in the terror-stricken grass, murmuring in his wicked heart, 'What more does he want of me? What else can he teach me? Have I not experienced the moment of eternity? Am I not Man and Man's comprehension? Am I not conscious of being Himself? Do I not finally have the certitude of being Love?'

"The deplorable effect of the first lie was to make us judge nature herself cruel and ungrateful, when in fact, projection of an interior world which is all emotion, she should have continued to appear to us even today full of charm, force, and clemency. The lie was born in the same instant that man ceased to feel himself in direct rapport with nature; for it is in judging worldly things by the nature of his fellow creatures that man acquired a false idea of good and evil. Evil exists only in man, and it is only through an absurd and disastrous extension that we have arrived at the shameful idea of evil as a natural principle. The study of his neighbor has led man to the bitter knowledge of his personality. That gloomy examination gave him a thousand reasons to mistrust his own soul; and from the moment he began to suspect the inner world of love, he regarded as vain, cruel, and ugly the exterior world that in sacred reality is subject only to the laws of beauty and harmony. Alas! What do we know today of nature? Do the least perverted among us know anything other than certain charms suitable at best only for gratifying the senses? Whatever we do, a feeling of regret is always part of the sad, aging love that we feel for this eternally young and passionate sister. Let us look around us: everything exudes vigor, confidence; the universe exults with tremendous desire; struggle is all, the struggle for love; power is all, and the right of the strongest love is the best. The soul of primitive heroes sings with the ocean, laughs with the torrent, and sobs with the breeze. Your soul recalls those songs, that laughter, those laments, and you look sadly out to sea and you sigh: 'Past, where are you, where are you? O my dear past, O my profound love buried forever!' Then you console yourself with some shameful sarcasm for the great misfortune of no longer being what you were at the beginning of time. The sun shines like an army drunk with victory; the blond beach shimmers like a beautiful body bathed with sensual delight; and wave follows upon wave, fleeting and tender image of love transitory and ever-present.

"A few steps from where you are, a pale and nervous dreamer, dead to love and combat, sighs weakly in the great striking sun: 'Why are things of so little reality so beautiful? Why this eternal invitation to the dance of life when in the night of my flesh, life waits only to forget having existed? How empty and flat am I, how patient and dull! How I have been duped, and what a horrible liar I am!'—And you, chevalier, and that great ninny, and I myself, are we not the least impure of all? Is it not a shame that idle curiosity about natural laws can take precedence over the mystical love of the universe? Consistently opposing the amorous invitation of sweet nature with a distrust engendered by a purely human lie; ceaselessly imagining some absurd discord between our senses and external events; unaware of the principle of the word and of the object, of that manifest love inherent in sky and sea, tree and wind, stone and heart;

unkind to our fellows, cruel to ourselves, in the heart of the most holy reality of God we live in an imaginary world of deceptions and illusions. Alas! A single word sufficed to destroy the august harmony that reigned on the first day between the two worlds of love and beauty. Think, chevalier! Man has just lied to man, his brother! Horrible moment! Termination, collapse, annihilation of everything! Man has lied to us, brother has deceived brother! Henceforth everything lies to you—God who created you for love, the beauty of heaven that commands you to love, and the holiness of the animal that licks your hand. All is destroyed, everything is pulled down. You shudder, your sight is veiled, the earth falls away under your footstep. Horror, ultimate horror! You feel the heartbeat of horror itself rise from the utmost depths of your being!"

At this point I could not stop myself from interrupting the count-duke with a gesture and a smile whose meaning did not escape the spirited inventor of paradoxes.

"So, then, monsieur le chevalier, it would appear that my remarks on the subject of falsehood are inadequate to convince you! Therefore I am constrained to commence a new digression, this time a little against my will. Nevertheless, I shall try to shed some light on my assertion. My reflections on the simultaneously tender and perverse nature of Annalena led me to doubt the moral equilibrium of my mistress. I then conducted the most detailed examination of this spirit of contradiction and falsehood with which my dearest appeared to be infused, and ended by establishing for all forms of alienation two perfectly distinct phases. This result of long study did not seem to me at all useless in an age in which the disciples of Aristotle rivaled those of

Hippocrates in ardor as they searched for the boundaries of responsibility. Any deviation of understanding is, if not preceded, at least accompanied by a more or less perceptible physical disorder in some part of the brain; from this simple fact it appears that every onset of madness must be conscious to a certain degree. Once the awareness of illness is admitted, at least in the first signs of derangement, we can do no less than attribute all maladies of reason to a division of the personality. Falsehood, the prime cause of these disconcerting sicknesses, is also the predominant character of their first stage. Woe to the man whose profaning word lies to the remnants of divine spirit that Heaven has left him! In him the perfect equilibrium of mind and matter is sundered forever. The liar has ceased to be the supreme expression of the affinity of substance and sentiment, of body and soul, of the interior world of love and the exterior universe of beauty. Truth survives still in the depths of his spiritual being; but already its appearance in the visible world has become doubtful. At the same time liar, negator of fact, and conscious of the truth, he himself is true and false in the same moment, and that moment marks the inception of a henceforth irreparable division of the personality.

"There you have, moreover, the reason why the simulation of health plays such an important part at the beginning of all psychic troubles. The sick person understands completely the menace which threatens him from his inner self; he feels himself becoming more of a danger to his fellow men with each passing hour; and yet pride and the fear of admitting his illness impose a criminal silence upon him. From that time on, his sole preoccupation will be to flee the infernal Double residing in his dark soul; he will find ingenious ways to deceive whoever approaches him as to the real state of his lamentable spirit ruined by falsehood. Before long he will demean himself to the point of hoping for salvation from the evil principle which was responsible for its loss. So the demented person remains aware of and accountable for his actions until the moment when the first stage of his illness gives way to either the rage of the manic or the profound exhaustion of the depressive. Most of our thieves, our assassins, and our politicians belong to the category of lunatics of the first degree. Profoundly steeped in the spirit of falsehood, most of the time they display, in their sinister undertakings, a power of dissimulation, a logic of probabilities, and a facility of execution of which sane men, that is, those who are loving and pious, seem to me to be absolutely incapable. In addition, the dreadful division of the personality never fails to extend its influence even to the structure of our bodies; for what the mind perceives as falsehood and transgression of the law of love becomes, to the flesh, vice and the sin of ugliness. As soon as duplicity intrudes on that which belongs to love, sensuality separates itself from the sentiment which made it an attribute of God, and material disintegration hastens moral division. It is therefore only half true to say that debauchery—by which I mean fornication without love—leads to madness; because vice is simply the consequence and the physical sign of the sin of falsehood, the only one which is mortal and unpardonable. ('All sins shall be pardoned, but the sin against the Spirit of truth never shall be pardoned.')

"Falsehood has so successfully poisoned the very principle of things that there is not one among us who can flatter himself that never has he heard fall from the lips of his love the word erased from the book of the world, the unique and very simple word whose absence was sufficient to render forever unintelligible the parable of life. This magical word is not a word of truth (according to the world's reality), as reality does not exist for the very simple reason that spirits filled with love would not know what to do with it. Nevertheless, if it is not truth to our minds, it is a veracity for our feelings, a veracity, a concern for accuracy which, in the spiritual order, is the very expression of the laws of matter. If you say: 'I love' when your heart is indifferent; or, 'I see,' or 'I feel,' when your eyes are in darkness or your senses deep in sleep, you cause an irremediable deviation in the natural order; the sharp, rasping grain of sand that is falsehood insinuates itself into the most sensitive cogwheels of the brain, and instantly you become to yourself an object without name, a word without meaning, a thing which exists and does not exist at the same time. The great, the awful calamity is to believe oneself a skeptic when one is simply a liar. Stupidly we mock that which in ourselves would be holy and real if we did not lack the force to discover the thousandth part of it in our neighbor. In his profound wickedness man has so acted that there is an aftertaste of poison in the healthiest food, and it is extremely difficult to separate the idea of love from that of good and evil; while in a world where falsehood remained the only unpardonable sin, the most extravagant show of affection would still elicit pardon for its naïveté; for there is no other way of measuring the moral value of our love or its object than the depth and truth of our feeling. Attachment to the created leads us to the love of the Uncreated; in loving well that which is limited, we lift ourselves unconsciously to supreme wisdom, infinite and beyond our understanding; thus, in the *Imitation,* the love of God personified is raised to the adoration of Love itself, of Love as the essence of life and the principle of being. Alas! what have we made of the charming, profound paradise of life? We who know, however, the task so simple, so sweet, incumbent upon us, we who feel that there is no object apart from Beauty, and no subject apart from Love; we who know, in a word, that any lie is comparable to those dark and distorted mirrors which receive beauty and give back ugliness! How I despise that blind enemy of divine reality, that black lie, prince of darkness, timorous, cringing repudiator of fact, of the naive and simple fact suffused with love! And how I should hate him, that dark lover of ugliness and decay, if I were able to despise him less! Each time that la Sulmerre opened her mouth and I caught on her face that simultaneously audacious and suspicious expression which precedes a lie, a secret voice cried out from the depths of my being: 'Take care, Pinamonte! By St. George, take care! The cavern yawns! The dragon is near, very near. . . . The world is already old and mildewed and worm-eaten; you yourself, despite your great love, so terrible and sweet, you are no more than the shadow of a dream, the memory of a vision which has vanished. Another lie, another sin against love, and all that which is tottering crumbles, and all that which is only appearance sinks forever into the impossible, into nothingness.' 'Stop, my beauty!' I cried then. 'Enough. Leave in peace those tender sentiments which are not yours. Tremble, madame, tremble, I tell you. The vengeance of Truth will be terrible, and how much more terrible the flash of lucidity which lies in wait for the madman on the brink of the tomb!' I pressed my hand against the beloved, despised lips, and at once the horrible serpent metamorphosed into a bird cooing with laughter—and what laughter!—with the silvery, roguish, carefree, absurd, and delicious laugh of my childhood! 'Look who's on his favorite topic again! Nevertheless, I need to speak to you very seriously, monsieur madman!'—'Never mind, madame liar. There is the spinet: go to the spinet or the harpsichord at once!'—And she ran merrily either to her spinet or to her harpsichord.

"She played these instruments ravishingly, and the preference she demonstrated for the works of Willibald Gluck gratified most pleasingly my taste for simple, mystical art. Our profound affection for music was perhaps the only spiritual bond between us. That divine art is the natural language of passion, the secret significance of tender or terrible accents overheard in the voice of the sea, the forest, the river, and the wind; and it is at the same time, in the dark, murky heart of our old race, the primitive, distinct echo of a forgotten harmony. Music is the cry of Love; Poetry is its thought. . . . One is the exaltation of the present and sings, 'I live and I love'; the other is the intoxication of memory which, when it proposes to express a love that is very real and full of life, seems to say, 'I have lived, I have loved. . . .' And that is doubtless the reason for which the two noble sisters, at first united in a single art, had to separate with the progress of time. . . . I loved to distraction Annalena's touch. As surprising as was the skill she displayed, never did I find a reason to doubt the sincerity of her emotion. The lovely musician was possessed of a very sensitive soul and the agility of her angelic hands had nothing in common with the irritating and vulgar dexterity of virtuosi. Her noble, mysterious visage reflected all the movements of passion, her dark eyelids fluttered voluptuously with the breath of harmony, yet her body never gave way to the ridiculous fits and starts of theatrical hysteria, nor did her charming head become disheveled by the winds of artificial tempests.

"Ah, chevalier, the memory of those plaintive, resonant hours moves me to tears! I lost Annalena and I lost music. While my beloved played, I lived outside of time; today, in the rhythm of the noblest works I hear only the footstep of death measured by the sterile tick-tock of clocks, and the instruments sound to my ear like empty tombs beneath the feet of the solitary stroller, or, under his stick, the large bones, rough and greenish, of cattle devoured by wolves, there in the country of my youth and of the handsome Stanislas.* Annalena at the harpsichord! Precious instants gone forever! I adore them, those unreal, supreme moments, all the more because they were always meted out to me with singular parsimony. You would have said of Annalena that she sought in music the expression of the greatest sincerity and purity of which her poor mortal heart was capable. Rarely would she approach her precious instruments without bestowing upon me a mischievous smile and words full of a cryptic playfulness. I have no recollection of ever having heard her play a single note in the presence of a third person. Some of those who admired her talent were astonished by the decision she seemed to have taken to cultivate it henceforth for the pleasure of only one person. As for Labounoff and the old duke of B———, they never lost an occasion to reproach her openly, but prayers, like laughter and sulks, were never able to overcome her amiable obstinacy; it even happened that one evening, in the midst of an eagerly attentive circle of music lovers, I heard fall from those sweet lips a retort whose boldness surprised me. 'Peace, messieurs; peace, for pity's sake; music itself would be but another affectation in this palace where truth and tenderness have no dominion; and it would be too much, truly, with the lie of my gaiety, my dancing, and my flowers.'

"What do you make of this, chevalier? Would not art be, to the liars that we are, a way of expressing indirectly the most urgent truths? . . . In any case, those noble evenings of music have left a most agreeable memory. As soon as Annalena opened her harpsichord, I hurried to light the candles and bolt the door, then went to curl up like a cat in my favorite corner beneath the sun and rain of Hogarth's *The Shrimp Girl*. Annalena struck the first chords; the tenuous tranquility of the chamber was filled at once with pensive music as well as with a fairylike perfume. The wall opposite looked at me through the empty masks of a Pietro Longhi canvas, the deathly pale masks of the *Women at the Menagerie*.* I was very fond of these nocturnal characters in courtly costumes gathered around an enigmatic buffalo. There is the buffalo, who is watching, and the remarkable ladies who are also watching; it is absurd, certainly; who would dare to dispute it? For after all, I ask you, why this menagerie, and why these masks, and why this motionless horned beast? But that is precisely a sufficient motive for these dreadful, wan creatures: they have nothing to say to you, absolutely nothing, and that is why your mind begins to question. Who are you, then, masks of Pietro Longhi? No answer. Who are you, bull so full of importance, and what the deuce are you doing there? Silence . . .

And who then am I, I who look at you contemplating a thing which doesn't exist? (Now do you perceive the reason for this fancy dress menagerie, monsieur le chevalier?) Yes, by the great devil of hell, who then am I in this dark corner? Why that animal, why this room, and why the masks, and Annalena, and myself, and this music and this night, this great deep night there over the roofs and over the waters? Is it the harpsichord tinkling or, under the hands of the queen of my soul, gold chiming, the golden harp of that beloved hair? Soft tinkle of the discreet harpsichord, of the singing furniture where all the secrets of my love, all the dusty, broken flowers of my memory sleep in love letters yellow with age. . . . A bit of Longhi for my passion for mystery, a little Hogarth for my cruel pity, a little—so little—of Annalena for my love of love, and I am alive! Very much alive! Not like that Pinamonte, that mime of life that I was once upon a time on the world's stage, perpetually astonished at being little more than a phantom, touching the silk of his breeches or the gold buttons of his jacket in the middle of the street, in the midst of a crowd, in order to truly convince himself of his materiality! Not like that Antisthène of posts and inns, confessor of the autumn winds and of the beggars of London Bridge, confidant of philosopher kings and consoler of deposed favorites. Ah! not like him, but alive, enamored of himself, huddled in a hard corner of the palace of amorous Certitude, a jealous, suspicious graybeard, no doubt deceived, loved a little for himself, a lot for his generosity; happy, happy in spite of everything, lulled by the most profound music, mocked by the most mysterious of beauties, sad and exuberant, ugly and handsome, shaken by a thousand shudders of astonished joy, and punctuating each of the master's phrases with a sigh containing all the nostalgia in the world. Tinkle, tinkle, tinkle, so sweet, so sad, so pure, so beautiful! still and forever!

"The marble slab offering little warmth to my backside, I went on tiptoe to look for a certain mauve silk cushion; then, blissfully sitting down again in my arcadian corner, I noiselessly stretched out my legs. . . . here again was one of my favorite spectacles: my spindly legs, those of a traveler with no destination! I gazed at them with love, those old legs of a great venturesome hare, I caressed them with a sympathetic hand; their shadow had marked off all the wearisome roads of the earth! And now the fairy of Music herself came on her feet of antique silk to bend over the dusty, cracked gaiters: the fairy of Music, monsieur le chevalier! The fairy of Music spoke tender words to my fossilized calves of an errant madman! 'Do you recall, noble legs' (I quote word for word), 'do you recall the damp grass trodden upon in former days at Marlow on the banks of a misty river criss-crossed by gray swans? Have you any recollection, O travelers, of the mossy echo which slumbers at Windsor, slumbers and speaks so softly in dreams? Will you once again slip on the yellow mud of the Warsaw Ghetto? How far away are the doorways of the Italian quarter of Dresden! O impatient, superb shadow! The imperial waters of the Neva know you, the colorless lakes of Muscovy remember you, the boulders of the Carpathians and the stones of the North Sea breathe your name in their dreams. What were you searching for, dashing about as you do? Roads, plains, footpaths, streets, and canals, London and Saint Petersburg! What have you found, rushing about and searching in that fashion?'

"With the gesture of Caesar astounded by the extent of the Empire's horizons, I naively showed it Clarice-Annalena. . . . Thereupon an incense shimmering with melodies was diffused throughout the chamber, a lulling ether of music, a breath of all the laughter of disenchantment and scorn, a cloud of all the sighs of sadness and love. . . . Lamps were going out somewhere very far away in the mists of the weeping night, so distant, so distant, farther away than the remotest seas . . . Strange crowds from times past swarmed before my eyes. Longhi's ladies took off their masks, the wall seemed naked to me . . . My head nodded a bit . . . Another note . . . another gust of wind against the window . . . I stretched out my traveler's legs . . . Another gleam of hair the gold of the plangent harp of Orpheus . . . and Pinamonte fell asleep in the melancholy of happiness.

"Such were the loves of our gallant shepherd: tender and rare, ridiculous and lamentable. Nothing, moreover, was more indicative of this peculiar oddness than my tragic obstinacy in aggravating a trouble of which I felt myself dying. In terror I watched the moment approaching when well-founded suspicions and real reasons for torment would no longer suffice for my senses blunted by grief and anguish. The thought to which I had come, that sooner or later I would have to give up my delicious torture, redoubled my ardor in researching the unknown elements of love. My soul became a secret and fearsome place: I enclosed myself therein with the dear obsessional phantom and the adorable *idée fixe* of my passion; with wise patience I elaborated therein the sentiment of the philosopher's stone, the elixir of perfect pain that was to immortalize my voluptuous martyrdom. I created new, undreamt of problems, puerile and cunningly tormenting; extravagant qualms, detailed and gnawing; strange composites of hellish lasciviousness and seraphic sentimentality. Tortured by hate, martyred by love, I had come to believe that I had dealings with demons as much as with angels, and I linked the image both adored and execrated of my love sometimes with the dreadful teraphim* of the Kabbalists and sometimes with the immaculate inhabitant of the supreme spheres of Swedenborg. At other times I consigned to paper the cries of my distress and the sighs of my amorous reveries. . . . Have mercy, monsieur le chevalier, let us leave in peace these pitiful nothings of yesteryear; do not press me to acquaint you with them. It is only too true to say that they were written with a pen dipped in the Phlegethon;* however, I prefer to leave to your imagination the task of creating an image of the joys and the torments of my passion. I deem it prudent, when one undertakes to bare his soul, to exercise the strictest control over his memory and his imagination; for it is unusual in such cases for expression to be subservient to truth. No matter what he does, the amorous narrator will always say more than he needs to; and no matter how little he gives rein to his fantasy, his tale will be engulfed by pathos. Most of the time in such cases innuendo is sufficient. Imagine, therefore, your own heart overflowing with tender and fierce passions, and then decant that amorous lava into the heart of the last Brettinoro: that is the surest means of forming an even slightly precise idea of my raptures and my sufferings. Particularly of the latter, alas! For I never tired of keeping alive in my heart the dark flame that devoured it; I was famished for sensual pleasure and for torment, and my hate was the equal of my love. Yes, I hated my dear mistress; I saw her dead in my dreams; her foul, putrid cadaver, filled with pus and bloated, swam in the midst of a river of filth: winged crocodiles, diseased and mucilaginous; paralyzed, deflated toads, glowing with the poisonous sweat of scrofulae; gigantic half-crushed insects, scaly, pustular, hairy, and greasy: all the most hideous monsters of fable and of fever took turns violating the liquefaction of the adored cadaver!

"My unhappy brain became the nocturnal rendezvous of the most dissolute company: riddled dandies carried on there disgustingly with their nauseating pock-marked goddesses; corpulent monks, pimply and boisterous, gorged with the flesh of their own bastards, drowned the remorse of their greedy paternity in wines concocted of the menstrual flux of female devils and of nuns' milk; concupiscent goats bedecked with lace head-dresses and poisoned banderillas paid violent court to the passivity of magnificent, sprightly popes of the Renaissance; pallid, dank polycephalic fetuses sometimes embellished these spirited and melancholy sessions with their childish gambols; while a horrible Clarice-Annalena, empress of the Gaupes★ and queen of Lesbos, invariably stretched out on a viscous mound of blind vermin and young eviscerated female lovers, presided from the height of her excremental, bloody throne over the lugubrious visions of my weakened brain.

"Moreover, the unspeakable preoccupations of my waking hours had little to envy in the dreams of my ignominious nights. My awakenings above all would have seemed to you distressing and grotesque beyond measure. First I directed venomous looks at my still-sleeping mistress: the flat, vaporous odor of her hair often repelled me; the sight of certain of her limbs made me shudder; and always the immobility of her slumber made me think of death. In one abrupt, desperate leap I left the amorous bed and bathed my pitiful head and all of my fanatic's body with fresh water; sighing, I swallowed a few drops of Hoffman★ and then a poor cup of chocolate and three or four slices of bread and butter. Then, going to Manto's bedside, I tore the beauty from the arms of Morpheus by means of insinuating, ingratiating caresses in which in turn my fingers, like those of a playful murderer, or my jaws, like those of an amorous hyena, seized her dazzling, graceful swan's neck. As innocent as these simulated strangulations were, they did not fail to result in extremely brusque and terror-stricken awakenings. Annalena's huge eyes opened without warning (you would have said, dear chevalier, two aloes of Tenarus wrenching themselves out of an age-old nightmare); terrified serpents rose up in the goddess's hair; and while a most disturbing shudder shook her lithe and delicate body, the too-well-loved minx clasped her clever little hands and plaintively cried out, 'O cruel friend! O barbarous lover! When will you cease to torment the gentle companion of your days? Do you think it so amusing to put the finishing touches on the bloody work of Cupid's arrows with the claws of cruelty?'

"These excessive preoccupations, these sorrows of soul and flesh, were often joined by worries of a more vulgar kind; for the uneasy love of the solitary and the jealous cannot help but resemble in certain respects the calculated and reluctant generosity of the avaricious. My enchantress, who certainly was not lacking in intelligence, had understood perfectly the nature of my feelings and had measured the depth of my love. Her vanity could not remain unaware of the blind adoration of a lover whose

127

renowned intellect equaled his illustrious birth; she knew the price of the sacrifices that I made each day for the sole purpose of assuring myself of her attachment and her fidelity; and I did not doubt that in the transports with which she returned my tenderness there was at least as much gratitude as sensual fancy. Her astonishment at the violence of my passion and the proud joy she derived from it often lent her visage a triumphant air which enhanced in my eyes its nobility and brilliance. My inflamed imagination observed my mistress' charms flower more each day; as my rapturous joy grew in the same degree, I soon began to consider Annalena's beauty as a work of my flesh and my mind, like a treasure painfully amassed through my efforts. On the other hand, my love often caused me great embarrassment, for la Sulmerre adored living with distinction and could not abstain from the world's glory. The attendance at the receptions she gave was as a rule quite high, and although I indulged her smallest wish she had never known the meaning of economy.

"Sincere affections are no freer of cost in this world than are venal loves, and the deepest devotion can triumph only with great difficulty over the habit of luxury and the taste for ostentation. In short, things came to the point where I often found myself constrained, in the midst of the most acute anguishes of love and jealousy, to venture into calculations whose figures, traced by a hand trembling with passion, lost themselves in manuscripts of poems inspired by the most extravagant of Muses. Sometimes my tragicomic, demented alarms were mingled with the cares a thousand times more laughable yet of a reasonable man. I trembled like a vulgar, ridiculous gallant, profiting from one of those stupid abandons common to beautiful women, profaning with one stroke the idol of my love and the altar of my sacrifices; my passion rose on occasion to the noble blindness of an author for his work, and yet I felt basely jealous of my generosity. I lost myself also in vain efforts to maintain my equilibrium, more hesitant each day, between a heart which grew heavier and heavier and a purse which grew lighter by the hour. The contradictory thoughts turning constantly in my mind often gave me the impression of originating in some obscure colloquy, absurd and passionate, between the most anxious Harpagon* and the touchiest Moor of Venice.

"On the days when there were large gatherings at the Riva dell'Olio I slipped away from la Mérone's residence and went off to bury myself in the humid darkness of my Barozzi burrow. There I found again my companions of the past, taciturn witnesses of an adventurous life: the ancient Giovanni with his wizened face, in a livery of spider webs; long missives scented with moss and tears, confidences of friends long since lost, forgotten, or dead; faded manuscripts full of yellowed scribblings, illustrated shrouds of a stillborn ambition; the poor portrait of Benjamin, yes, chevalier, the poor flaking portrait of Benjamin, stolen one evening from Manto and carried lovingly against my heart; expired passports, detailed and suspect, with the eagles of Prussia and of Russia; the snuffbox of Stanislas,* the little knife, carver of initials and hearts, souvenir of the forty-year-old on the Ile Saint-Louis; the lid of the box where, as a child, I had tried to draw the chateau of Brettinoro with its park, Don Quixote's willow tree, the mossy bench and the romantic fountain. . . .

"Wretched objects of bygone days! With what morose

delight I inhaled their commingled odors of fruit and the grave, of April rain and mice, of dreams and reality! How well they had portrayed, in time past, that great child's love that lived on now in my old man's heart, the fabulous flower that bloomed in the garden of innocence! With what tender disdain I reread all those introductions, meditations, objections, remarks! Innocent jumble of emotions clumsily disguised as reasonable arguments, of biases learnedly presented as deductions, nakedness of soul daubed with spangles of wit! And how everything that proceeded from my life as a man seemed dark and mean, but clear and profound when it came from my life as a child! Love, love! O master of the celestial realm of Simplicity! I spread out all these souvenirs on a table; I contemplated them, turned them over again and again, coaxed them; I spoke to them, gently made fun of them . . . In truth, chevalier, in the heart of joy nothing is sweeter than to regret sadness!

"On a day when I idled like this among familiar objects, I took it into my head to go to see the lady Gualdrada in her garret. Despite the curiosity which my peculiar hostess inspired in me, until now I had limited my contacts with her to the exchange of courteous salutations in the street or on the stairs; Giovanni, with his curiosity about everything, visited her often and knew her well enough to have set her gossiping, and he never tired of laughingly reproaching my indifference to her place. Having resolved therefore to end this refrain once and for all, I took courage and bounded up the spiral staircase that led to the old woman's cubbyhole. I found the wicked fairy Carabossa, spectacles on her nose, shivering, huddled in a rickety armchair and bent over a voluminous treatise on demonology. Upon seeing me she rose with an air of haste and bowed to me. An open smile immediately lit up her sad face, yellowed and covered with warts, her gray, watery eyes unnaturally enlarged by the double lenses which shaded them. She humbly carried to her trembling lips the hand I extended to her, and her ceremonious phrases uttered in a soft, quavering voice seemed to come from the depths of another century. A rapid look around her dismal abode enlightened me as to the life and tastes of the old woman. The three damp and gloomy rooms of which it consisted were an arena for the cavortings of a large muddy toad, a black cat, and a crippled hen of the same color that continuously hopped about on furniture no less touching than she herself. A great armoire with a glass door showed a confused heap of dusty, bizarre objects such as caskets made of red or yellow wood curiously carved, Huron headdresses bristling with feathers of a hundred colors, clubs painted by island savages, ancient arms of Spanish manufacture, and a thousand other objects I could not name. It was not long before the chattering of my hostess revealed the key to all this mystery. In her youth, the poor hunchback had been foolish enough to listen to the compliments and boasts of a tall adventurer who was only after the tidy dowry which he knew she possessed. Gualdrada being an orphan, and the devil taking a hand in the affair, the marriage soon took place. Not long after the ceremony Sciancato, the young bridegroom, makes the acquaintance of a band of escaped convicts who disclose to him their fine plans of piracy and treasure-hunting. Sciancato, tired of living indolently off the infirm girl, agrees at once and allows himself to be presented as a captain. A casket disappears from Gualdrada's chest, a sailing vessel is chartered, and our gallant adventurer is now a buccaneer. The unfortunate Gualdrada, madly enamored of her rogue, entreats him, tears out her hair, fills the air with prayers and lamentations . . . in vain! The mast is raised, the unfeeling Sciancato embarks. 'Is everything in readiness? Let's go!' He gives the signal, he departs, he is gone. And the lady Gualdrada is abandoned, hopeless, and half-ruined besides: only the Barozzi home remains of her respectable fortune. After reading the cards over and over for herself, she conceives the idea of becoming a soothsayer. The ungrateful Sciancato unexpectedly reappears one fine day, however, laden with rich booty and exotic gifts. A week of delirious joy . . . and he is gone again. Ten years, fifteen years, twenty years. . . The small body becomes frail, the hump rounder, the beautiful hair of the ugly woman turns gray under her lace caps . . . Alas! lost forever. Not a sign of life . . . In what deep, bitter, wild waters lie his bleached old bones? Against what purple horizon of mourning does his skeleton of a nameless hanged man swing?

"During this entire recital (which lady Gualdrada, with visible pleasure, prolonged to excess), I experienced difficulty in restraining the satanic laugh that choked me and the irksome tears with which compassion filled my eyes . . . So then, I said to myself, does that terrible, sweet love make a game of pursuing me ceaselessly in its noblest or its most appalling aspects? Wherever I walk, a secret spring always causes a little monster with the head of a god or of a devil to erupt from below the earth! It rules my thoughts, it governs the world. It is here, it is there! Here, there, over there, farther away, everywhere! The invisible threads that control the motley marionette of the universe knot themselves around the little claw of the wheedling, cruel traitor. He tugs: the satellite flits frantically around his astral flower; the turbulent tide swells with a thousand impatient bosoms; the sap rumbles, the blood catches fire, the seed cries toward the light; the arms of prayer lift to heaven; all the womb, all the flesh of the earth is in labor! He tugs, the scoundrel, he tugs! Tender Philomel's* throat blows the bubbles of her soul in the colors of tears and blood; the amorous viper leaves her horrible hole, rises up and comes to prick up her avid ear; the breeze wakes, the pollen takes flight in downy, fecund kisses; the ladybug lights her lantern; the water spider at the heart of the water lily pursues his hairy beloved; the bard tunes his lute in the North tower; Pinamonte presses both hands to his rapidly beating mad heart; and lady Gualdrada, a silvery scarf over her bouncing hump, runs to the window to look toward the indistinct old port through the telescope of the buccaneer she will never see again . . . Never? Ah, never, alas!

"And with heavy-hearted astonishment mixed as much with disgust as with pity, I contemplated the ancient abandoned woman so ridiculous and so doleful. 'Who would have thought,' spoke the little gray lips, dessicated and trembling, 'who would have suspected, monsieur? After a honeymoon so tender, so passionate! For he really loved me, oh! I'm certain of it, he really loved me and he still loves me, yes, yes.' And the little witch's head nodded 'yes, yes,' and the large hump nodded 'yes, yes,' and all of the small pitiful body of a hospital doll nodded 'yes, yes' also, with a rustling of the skeleton of a bird, of a frozen shrub, of a dusty little stuffed creature that dances on the wall when the air moves. O Love, O cruel Love, what are you doing here? Answer, it is Pinamonte, your faithful follower, your devotee, who speaks to you! O Love, what are you doing here? And the Immense, the Impenetrable, the Terrible, the Gentle One answered me with the tears and sighs of the unfortunate woman: 'I am here because I am everywhere. I am grief and joy, hope and memory; I am here because I am the Moment, the great Moment of eternity. I am in Gualdrada because Gualdrada is a thing, because I am in all things, because all things are in me. I am Beauty and Adoration, Sorrow and Pity; in heaven I am the sublime Father of all and on earth I am the Son, stoned, bloody, covered with spittle. And in your heart I am that which desires, and the great silent night, cold and deaf on the Mount of Olives, and the cross whose shadow covers the earth, the universal Dominations and the unending Resurrection. I am the blind man's eye, the ear of the deaf, and when I appear to the weeping sister in my true form, the brother rises from the coffin.'

"Gualdrada's secret certainly was surprising in itself, but when the old woman assured me that she had never breathed a word of it to anyone, not even to my old servant, I found even stranger the realization that she considered me such a close friend. At first I could not understand why the necromancer had chosen me for her confidant; soon, however, I realized that love had divined love, and that underneath the open conversation between the coxcomb and the old woman there ran the secret murmur of a dialogue between Sciancato and Annalena. Only quasi-confessions choose the wrong confidant; complete sincerity, amorous sincerity, always speaks to the one who knows it, who loves it, and who expects it. The thirteenth sovereign prince of Brettinoro received the confession of lady Gualdrada, which definitely was not lacking in either charm or grandeur. While listening to the witch's jeremiads I intently examined the image of our bizarre group reflected in a tall mirror. Everything was as it should have been in the scene offered to my view: perfect harmony, physical and moral, reigned; and the setting was wondrously appropriate. In the light from a dim window filled with a hazy old sky, the little hunchback crouched in the hollow of an enormous unsteady, creaky armchair embroidered with yellowed birds, frayed flowers, patched little shepherds and shepherdesses; and on a ripped footstool facing her, Pinamonte, legs nonchalantly extended, chin on his sword-hilt. The splish, splash of the toad. The cluck, cluck, cluck of the hen. The purring of the cat. The armoire crammed full of the mute tumult of mementos; on the wall the disquieting gambols of three great immortal spiders and two graveyard woodlice, fat and heavy; old cards scattered here and there; everywhere dust and things beyond repair. Have you ever played in the damp corners of a neglected apartment with a little blonde girl who says, 'Let's not go there, for heaven's sake; the devil must be there'?

"Without warning I stiffened from head to toe with the desire to see Annalena naked amid this desolation and dust. Abruptly taking leave of the fortune-teller, I dashed off to find out from Giovanni the day and the hour when the witch left her lair. The factotum informed me that rarely did she miss a mass or a sermon, and that every Sunday he was in the habit of accompanying her to San Maurizio for vespers. It was a Friday: never was the Lord's Day awaited with more impatience. I confided my strange whim to Manto. At first she merely laughed, calling me a perverted old beau, but soon, after my description of the projected scene, her beautiful schoolgirl eyes filled with certain secret fires that could have shaken all the devils of hell. She even suggested to me that . . . And the fear of seeing the heavy bonnet and spectacles of the fairy Carabossa appear at any moment . . . There was only time for . . . Forgive, chevalier, these shocking details. . . .

"Surrounded as I was by real rivals and continuously haunted by imaginary traitors, I could not enjoy a single moment of hearts-ease or peace of mind, and my miserable days were wasted in waiting for the most terrible catastrophes and in planning the cruelest revenge. I constantly denounced all humanity; I cursed fate, the gods, creation, and, to the depths of my being, those who had conceived me. Nevertheless, in the worst of my suffering and my paroxysms, I felt in my secret flesh and soul a kind of dark and strange pleasure which seemed to be composed of titillating anguish and gnawing delight, and of which I can only give you some idea by comparing it to the mysterious and appalling emissions of the hanged. Even while abominating these shameful and sinister sensations I could not stop myself from ceaselessly inflaming their vile, painful barb. Plagued without respite by the most libidinous and most insane jealousies, I turned to trickery and, employing (God alone knows with what clumsiness!) the classic stratagem of unexpected departures, I would post myself in the most fantastic disguises to a particular corner of a dark street from which I could, without for the most part being disturbed by anyone, keep the melancholy old palace of my mistress under surveillance for hours. It would have been wiser without question to entrust my beauty to the care of some sensible duenna or to have her watched over by a band of nimble guards paid handsomely for their duties; but this vulgar method of assuring the fidelity of a lover was repugnant to an extravagant love whose object, however much a stranger to the virtues of angels, only seemed to me more endowed with the formidable charms that imagination attributes to the spirits of darkness.

"On the other hand, even while heaping imprecations upon love and upon the jealous suspicions which made my life a torture, there was nothing in the world I feared more than discovering a betrayal that perhaps would have delivered me from my torments forever; for like the majority of human beings, I preferred the illusion by which doubts are lulled over the disillusion that certainty brings. The innocent stratagem of nocturnal spying was the most natural thing in the world, with the double advantage it seemed to offer of pandering to my romantic tastes and, at the same time, sparing my heart the sorrows of a definitive disenchantment. It was both the most delicious irritant and the most benign remedy to my suffering. How exquisite a thing is emotion, even the most painful! Yes, monsieur le chevalier, I have the most vivid and tender memories of these transports of voluptuous mistrust; my disillusioned heart still loves them with all of the nostalgia experienced by an old ruined cardplayer recalling the precious anguish of three aces. Huddled in my damp hideout like an animal on the alert, or upright and frozen in the immobility of a saint nailed in his niche, my eyes passionately followed the movements of light and shadow in the rooms of my lovely one; I trembled at the faintest noise; the approach of a passerby woke painful echoes in my heart; I felt myself surrounded by dark mysteries, implacable hatreds, nameless perils.

Filled with timorous rage, I examined attentively the silent, gloomy alley: in each cavalier who crossed it I thought I recognized a rival, a base seducer; in each old woman walking by with a halting step, a loathsome procuress working to ruin me. The night enfolded me in its damp shadows; the autumnal rain and hail lashed my face; prophetic drunks poured abuse upon me; I remained indifferent to all insults.

"These ridiculous eccentricities astonish you, chevalier. They never ceased to surprise me as well. For—I cannot say it too often—the strange duality from which I suffered had in no way affected my reason, and the old circumspect and disenchanted Brettinoro never tired of reviling the new thoughtless, hotheaded Pinamonte, pointing out to him a hundred times a day the artlessness of his feelings and the coarseness of his dissolute habits. 'O insanely amorous graybeard, O most craven Benedetto, O most miserable Guidoguerra!' Thus he inveighed against me in the dark corner which served as the observation post for my overly suspicious passion. 'O most unfortunate dupe of love! What folly is yours! Do you not see the abyss that the most ridiculous blindness digs beneath your feet? You old cooing, featherless pigeon! Impetuous old fool! Go into yourself; perhaps there is still time! What will become of you, Pinamonte of the Devil, the day your purse, already much lighter, will be good only as a handkerchief for your watery nose or toilet paper for your yellow-bellied senile despair? Ah, by the Styx, is this the fruit of the wise counsels of M. de la Bretonne?* On your feet, Brettinoro! Friend of Lauraguais,* emulator of Briqueville,* shake off this torpor; your dreams are perfidious, and the worst afflictions lie in wait for you.'

"However, the jealous wretch remained deaf to the exhortations of reason and Brettinoro played the thankless role of a Cassandra to Pinamonte. As atrocious and ridiculous as my amorous anguish was, it never ceased to appear preferable to the horrible solitude of mind and heart that made me odious from the earliest recollections of my youth. In these interior conflicts, the advantage consistently remained with love, and even while scorning la Sulmerre, I sometimes caught myself entertaining the extravagant idea of assuring myself of possessing her completely by means of a legal union. Which only proves that the miserable human mind, pitiful compilation of obscure preconceptions, timid resignations, and specious judgments, always ends by surrendering to the stealthy, subtle persuasion of Sentiment, which is the essence itself and the only master of a subconscious humanity and of a world completely pervaded by a terrible and tender mystery.

"Moreover, the only result of all these mockeries and all these reproaches was always to needlessly exacerbate the feeling that I was weak and ridiculous. The rough, cutting wit of my morose joking cruelly reopened in my heart the fire of the wounds created there each day by passion. Powerless to cure my madness, these belated regrets were at best capable of reminding me of the risk I ran of losing myself in the world's opinion. I blushed at playing the role of a gloomy jealous lover in an intrigue where my frivolous rivals doubtless saw only the most vulgar farce; and along with everything else I feared that, wearying of the absurdities of the old beau, the malevolence of those surrounding me would reach the point of attacking the honor of a gentleman. The clash of so many conflicting emotions exceeded my reason. It amazed me that scorn and fear could occupy so much space in a heart filled with tenderness. To submit to the judgment of the world a passion that sometimes raised my soul to God was also more than a little repugnant to me, and I did not stop cursing my love except to reproach myself for my ingratitude. 'Lunatic!' I cried then, 'Lunatic! Will you allow yourself to be oppressed until the final day by the habit of falsehood and the tyranny of prejudice? Don't you know that the beloved being, bad or good, noble or contemptible, is never anything but a superficial apparition and that the end of every love is in the bosom of the unique Being? What does the fuel matter if the flame reaches up to heaven? Are you fearful of being mocked by the crowd of fools? The object of your flame is full of grace, how could you be ridiculous? Is it your own judgment that you fear? Your love is sincere; if the priest condemns it, what angel of true purity would dare even accuse it? No! I read something very different in your miserly old hypocrite's mind: the image of the poor young rival haunts your unhappy brain. In your miserable heart avarice competes with jealousy for first place. There is your ridicule, and there is your impurity.'

"The attitude of grandeur and defiance that accompanied these violent soliloquies, the arrogant, fierce image the mirrors reflected at those moments, the authoritarian sound of voice, the vivacity of gesture—everything seemed as if it must reinforce the eloquence of the words and reestablish at last calm in my soul . . . Alas! to my heart, nothing could equal the strange attraction of anxiety! After an hour or two of calm, jealous concerns took hold of me again and I trembled in my terror as the moth sputters in the deadly flame. Let it be said in my favor, however, that the world seemed to have taken it upon itself to nourish the anguish that devoured me. Stupid envy already circulated the most bizarre rumors about me: Giovanni reported a few which gave me grounds for serious reflection. As la Sulmerre was considered quite rich and I totally ruined, certain of my detractors accused me of living off my mistress, others that I intended to become the master, by means of a scandalous marriage, of her ill-gotten riches; some imbeciles went even farther, pushing their maliciousness to the point of suspecting both of us of criminal commerce with the princes of Friendship!

"Extremely irritated by these idiotic calumnies, I resorted to guile and strove to mislead the heraldic, scribbling mob that constituted la Mérone's entourage as to the true nature of my feelings. Without any doubt it was an extremely delicate undertaking, for the vulgar frequenter of palaces is harder to fool in worldly matters than the rabble of the streets. Nonetheless, my efforts were crowned with all the success of which I considered them worthy. Constantly applying myself to disguising my feelings, I lost no time in mastering the art of dissimulation, and soon had the satisfaction of reading on everyone's face the disappointment caused by the rapid cooling of a passion which they willingly imagined to be heavy with ludicrous disasters and fertile with scandals of more than one kind. Whatever scorn I felt for my entourage, I was amazed to discover not one who was at least capable of appreciating the skill which I demonstrated in feigning, in the extremes of my tragic passion, the outward appearance of a scoundrel in search of diverting, ephemeral adventures. Only my roguish enchantress divined the melancholy secret of my soul; she even seemed to me to be touched sometimes by a certain compassion, for the minx had a sensitive streak and lacked neither spirit nor heart. However, her tender feelings were of very brief duration and usually ended in an outburst of hysterical hilarity which in most cases I could not keep myself from echoing, so amusing did I find the contrast which I continuously discovered between my natural mood and the borrowed character of the part I played before the envious gallery.

"Thus I soon was obliged to understand that a gathering which so willingly permitted itself to be fooled was at the very most deserving of my contempt, and this thought was enough to make me disgusted with the too-easy success of my pretense. Moreover, it was not long before I saw in the cleverness of my simulation one more proof of the degeneration of my will, and in my persistence in concealing my atrocious anguish the gravest symptom of the illness in which it originated. I horrified myself, I took pity on both my heart and my soul; I felt my instinctive hatred of duplicity grow from hour to hour; my innocent affections appeared before me in the anxious fever of insomnia with the odious features of falsehood and madness; finally I became convinced that even the sense of honor had become foreign to me and that, beneath the disguise of these base displays of bravado, my weakness had been transformed into cowardliness. Nothing had ever tormented me more than this fear of losing the little energy remaining to me and becoming a docile marionette controlled by the charming, capricious fingers of a woman. Wherever I went, my silent obsession followed me like a faithful dog.

"You laugh, monsieur le chevalier; alas! Know then that my madness accompanied me everywhere in the form of a real dog! I had become subject to visions: not content with torturing my poor brain night and day, the ghastly *idée fixe* made my blood run cold by appearing to me in the repellent aspect of a starving, sniveling, mangy old cur . . . O, the small body covered with pustules, the thin paws, the hairless swollen rump, the scarlet organ in eternal erection, of this ill-humored specter, this foul dog of my soul! Insolent and somber image! I see it always before my eyes; time has not dimmed it, death will be powerless to erase it from my memory. Alas, no! When death comes, the bloated cadaver of the frightful animal will follow my boat along the Lethe. Each time that I turn back to this horrible epoch of my life, a shudder of revulsion shakes me from my peruke to my heels. The tomb arouses neither fear nor love. Eternity has nothing more to teach me.

"Revolted beyond measure by my double role of gay ladies' man and doleful lover, my mind endlessly devised a thousand vengeful plans to break off and decamp; however, whichever way I turned in the depths of my absurd despair, I found everywhere only the drawn nets of the traps set by love. What means of deliverance would I not have used in my laughable distress? To which vices would I not have appealed in this search for a distraction from my cowardly aberration? Toasting in champagne my victories, drowning in wine my losses at cards, I went from gambling house to cabaret and from cabaret to public bordello, hailed everywhere as king of the card tables and emperor of the tipplers. Where could one find the Scarron⋆ capable of describing the farcical exuberance of my bouts of drunkenness, the Hogarth worthy of painting the burlesque melancholy of my hours of remorse? How many times in the tumult of my thoughts did I escape in the night from the palace of la Mérone to run, hair flying in the wind, wild-eyed, filth on my lips, to wake the placid Giovanni, guardian of my house and confidant of my troubles? The streets are deserted, the canals sleep soundly. I run, I leap, I fly in the shadows. My frozen, withered arm waves an unlighted lantern. Love, jealousy, awareness of my ridiculousness, fear of dishonor, hatred of my unknown rivals pursue me like so many fiery little devils. Hare, antelope, I bound over steps, bridges, and barriers; bull, I break down the door of my house with blows of my head and my feet; finally, Antisthène and old fop, breathless, tearful, grumbling, exhausted, I fall into the paternal arms of my family's old servitor.

"'This is the end, I'm done for, Giovanni! I am alone, all alone in the world! Open your comforting arms to me! You, at least, spawn of the devil, would not have betrayed me! Do you know what it is to be alone, all alone in the world? Horror! Profound horror! Nonetheless, you must admire the generosity of my soul, the magnitude of my resolve, for we are leaving, Giovanni, we will pack up and go, we will abandon now and forever the hideous abode of stupidity, envy, and perfidy. We are heroes, we who bear the name of Brettinoro, San Benedetto, Guidoguerra of the first crusade . . . Well, then! it appears that you do not admire my calm, Giovanni so wise and faithful; however, my wrath is full of moderation and august majesty. O joy! the hour of vengeance has sounded. We are free! Free as a denizen of the air, independent as the soul of proud philosophers! Farewell, Venice, accursed city, padded cell of Italy! Let us break away, Giovanni; words are passé; we need, by God's blood, actions, only actions!'

"Without evincing the slightest astonishment or the least doubt as to my sudden decision, the discreet Giovanni, perfect connoisseur of the human heart, immediately went to work; and I, cursing all the while like a fine devil, helped him as best I could: books, clothing, boxes, and trinkets were merrily swallowed up by the voracious trunks. All was now ready, night was fading and, at the instant of closing the last bag, the rosy fingers of daybreak came to join ours. The dawn of the great day was there, monsieur le chevalier! Giovanni called porters, gave orders, negotiated with the gondoliers, inquired about ship sailings. My satanic laugh dominated the disputes, the songs, the laughter, the gibes; perched casually on an inverted piece of furniture, I assumed the airs of a conqueror, my whip became the baton of a marshal of France; I was coquettish about my misfortune; I gave unstintingly on all sides to rogues and rascals, I comforted lady Gualdrada, I felt powerful and victorious—imagine, chevalier! I had vanquished love, of all gods the most feared! At last the cautious Giovanni opened wide the doors and gave the signal to depart; the joyous caravan of porters followed in disorder; merry and bellicose, I brought up the rear. We descended to the street. Ah, chevalier, to the street! To the street, alas! . . . The city still pale with sleep, the silence, the scent of the water . . . Instantly I ceased my boasting and became once again the pitiful Pinamonte; the sadness of leaving clutched savagely at my heart, the awful phantom of my former solitude threatened me from under the bridges; the gaze of passersby, the colors of the sky, the smell of the wind, the lighted windows, all, all of them spoke to me of the agonizing solitude which awaited me there, somewhere, anywhere, far away, very far away. An avalanche of old snow, dirty and spongy, crushed my heart; the mournful sun of the past lit my memory; and each time that my thoughts returned to my cruel destiny, an absurd and repugnant image lurched across my soul: my wretched old abandoned dog, starving and scruffy. Heavens! how close was la Sulmerre! How far the China of her Benjamin! Annalena! Annalena! O the sweetness of accepting all humiliations! O the happiness of resigning oneself to sleep away his life of incredulity, renunciation, and boredom in the soothing, treacherous arms of Manto! Everything around me seemed dreary and miserable; I was ready to succumb under the terrible weight of the atmosphere, of the sky, of life . . . Turning with a piteous air toward my old valet, 'Giovanni,' I stammered, 'faithful Giovanni! You understand me; the human soul is nothing more than whim and weakness; you yourself, friend in knavery, do you not sometimes complain because your heart is too sensitive? Ah, Giovanni! What have we done? Where are we running? What demon is driving us away from here? Will we never find a shelter where our old vagabond bones can rest?' Giovanni pretended to turn a deaf ear to my plea and, followed by the cortege of bearers, calmly continued on his way. Head low, heart furiously reprimanding my body from the knees to the roots of my peruke, my blood frozen with cowardliness, my soul shamed to death, eyes burning with tears, I followed, reeling, the merry team of porters. Finally, anger and despair having made me shake off all false shame, with a terrifying look I gave my people the order to turn back. On the occasion of my first attempt at deliverance

I had the audacity to flee as far as Trieste; the second time, courage took me as far as the port; but after the third time I never found the strength of will to get past the corner of my street.

"Thus the old raven, broken of the habit of freedom, went back to his regular flight toward the adored and accursed cage, and never did a bird who had escaped and been beaten by the violent winds and rain of the seas taste more repentant joys or more tender endearments on its return. But these pure delights of reunion did not last long, for I returned to my suspicions and my rancors as one returns to sad, worn-out old friendships. Can the melancholy pleasures of our reconciliations be otherwise? More often my frivolous lover doled them out to me capriciously rather than according to the secret desire of her heart; and even when the fervent expression of her forgiving tenderness seemed to show less distrust or impatience, my ever-vigilant jealousy always interrupted the flow with some absurd outburst.

"I shall not expand upon our stupid, noisy quarrels; the memory of them that I have kept fills me with disgust and anguish, for sometimes they degenerated into veritable brawls in the course of which the amorous tyrant gave way to the captious torturer. A raging lust brought its arms to these shameful combats, and peace treaties were then sealed with tears, delight, and, sometimes, blood. Stealthy and taciturn respites usually followed these tempests of the heart and the senses; unfortunately I never knew how to use them except to deaden by means of useless quibbling the sensible regrets which tormented me; and, thus casting the entire burden of blame on the dear shoulders of my enchantress, it was not long before I became once more the prey of my suspicions and of my desires for flight and vengeance. To anyone but you, this condition would be inexplicable in a man completely aware of his weakness and yet ceaselessly involved in heroic projects of deliverance; but it is the folly of true devotees of love to seek bitter pleasure in those thoughts and feelings that seem to thwart them in the cruelest, surest manner in the world.

"The preoccupation of avenging an insult which, if not certain, is at least very probable, was not foreign to the antics of my enamored hatreds and my restive flights; nevertheless, it played only a secondary role. Certainly I took a malicious pleasure in imagining, during the preparations for a voyage, the scenes of surprise or of despair which my sudden disappearance would cause: the consternation, the despondency, the shame of la Mérone, the anger of her brother Alessandro, the astonishment of the young lap-dogs of her retinue, the jeers of the superannuated gallants of her court, the gossip of the church, the good spirits of Labounoff, the admiration, rather guileful and mixed with vexation, which the decisiveness of a nobleman sacrificing love to honor, happiness to pride, and pleasure to disdain, must inspire in my rivals. Whatever pleasure, however, I found in entertaining these vengeful images I forgot as soon as, the hour of supreme farewells sounding, unhappy reality ordered me to proceed from plan to execution; for charming and cruel nostalgia awaited me at the door of my house, the mournful flower of memory in its hand. I then abandoned myself to the somber joy of regret, to the mortal intoxication of despair; and I returned to my lamentable nature of Antisthène and of Pinamonte.

"My fine resolutions to break away were usually whispered by the voice of anger and of shame; nevertheless, they must have had an attraction stronger than vengeance itself, because, despite the pitiful result of my previous flights, I was unable to give up pursuing their realization. There is no question that vengeance is a kind of sensual pleasure and nothing, in my opinion, less resembles the love of justice; for when we resort to reprisals we are less concerned with offering an example of justice than with repaying our pain with the pleasure we experience in causing suffering in our turn. No matter how grave an insult, we never discover the motives except by means of an approximate reckoning, especially with respect to love; and there always remains some obscure point because no one can fathom completely the soul of the guilty person. On the other hand, however great a part in the act of vengeance we wish to assign to impulse, premeditation still remains a confirmed fact, with the result that the reasons for vengeance always appear to be clearer and surer than the motives for offense.

"My situation was more complex, however, for added to the desire to cause distress to la Sulmerre was the peculiar wish to torment my own heart. You already know, monsieur le chevalier, the sadness of my separations from Annalena. To crown my misfortune, or perhaps from an excess of ridiculousness, mourning for my love was accompanied by the absurd regret of people and especially of objects that were witness to my capricious happiness. 'Alas, Pinamonte, crazed old head!' I sighed foolishly in my heart, 'You will drag your vagabond footsteps along all the world's roads; but no matter what you do, solitary and nostalgic invoker, you will never again hear them echo in the rooms of your dear cruel one! This sky that arches over your head you will no doubt know, in your unhappiness, for a long time yet;

but never again will you contemplate it from the flowered old balcony of the House of Happiness. Do you recall how the gondoliers serenaded you last year under the windows of your love? You heard it while half-asleep, deep in the great antique bed perfumed with the dreams of the drowsing Annalena. Brettinoro of misfortune, Guidoguerra of the devil! And that dark little corner between the fireplace and the oak chest, where you went to nestle during the absences of your lover? With backside on the hard, cold marble of the paving stones, eyes lost in the false sky of the ceiling, and an uncut book in your hand, what delicious hours of melancholy and waiting you lived there, you old imbecile! The daylight died in the tall cloudy windows; twilight enfolded you in private, profound music; your heedless soul followed the flight of a large horsefly drunk on love and sleep, small bass voice of summer, minuscule spinning top of old Germany. To live and die in this corner of the sentimental chamber, you said to yourself; yes, to live and die there: why not, monsieur de Pinamonte, friend of dark and dusty little corners? Here lives the meditative spider, powerful and happy; here the past curls up and makes itself so small, an old ladybug seized with fear . . . Ironic, cunning ladybug, here the past rediscovers itself and remains undetectable to the learned spectacles of collectors of pretty things. Here you find a thousand cures for boredom and an infinity of things worthy of occupying your mind for all eternity: the musty odor of moments three centuries old; the secret meaning of the hieroglyphics of fly specks; the triumphal arch of this mouse hole; the fraying of the tapestry against which your round, bony back lounges; the rodent noise of your heels on the marble floor; the sound of your dusty sneeze, Leporello's song in falsetto; the soul, in a word, of all this ancient dust in a corner of the room forgotten by the feather duster . . . And you wept, old Pinamonte, really! You surprised yourself weeping . . . For as a child you already had a taste for the deserted attics of chateaux and unused library corners, and you avidly read without understanding a single word the Dutch privileges of the folios of Diafoirus★ . . . Ah, you rogue, the delicious hours that you passed, in your villainy, in the recesses sprinkled with nostalgia of the palazzo Mérone! How you wasted your time in penetrating to the soul of things which had made it their own! With what happiness you were transformed into an old lost slipper escaped from the gutter, rescued from the sweepings, into one of a pair of dice kicked there by the foot of a gambler a hundred years ago, into the head of a wooden doll forgotten in this corner of the room during the last century . . . The mystery of things, small sentiments in time, great void of eternity! All infinity found room in this stone corner, between the fireplace and the oak chest . . . Brettinoro! Guidoguerra! Where are they now, God's blood! Where are the great joys you took from a spider, your profound meditations on a spoiled, dead little thing? And that bedside rug, that melancholy bedside rug whose garden of wool engaged your somnolent mind when you awoke?

"'O San Benedetto! Pitiful lunatic enemy of your heart! Think of the lamp, the very old lamp, that greeted you from far away at the window of your thoughts, at the high window burned by ancient suns, which you called your Rowena★ . . . the trembling light of your lamp will be still from now on . . . What will it think of you, poor, treacherous, nervous soul, what will the familiar old lamp think of you during the nights of winter and desertion? What will they think of you, the things that were so dear to you, as dear as brothers? Was not their obscure destiny closely linked to yours? You gave much of your soul and imparted a little of your life to these humble objects; do you now wish to betray them, do you want to abandon them, plunge them back into their nothingness, you who were so tender yesterday, you who are so cruel today? Immobile, mute things never forget: melancholy, scorned, they receive the secret of what is most humble in us, most obscure deep inside us. O Pinamonte of the Devil! Your soul is much closer to things than it is to the unhappy self that you call your reason. Your reason! Frivolous enemy of silence, poor animated, noisy thing swollen with illusions and alarms! Think of objects, of dull, nameless objects, mute confidants of your love. They live longer than men; do not despise their silence, which is so old! It has so many things to say. You are leaving, Pinamonte; you are going far away, Brettinoro! You are escaping, Guidoguerra! Your madman's long legs and your impossible dreams carry you off; the tempest of your wrath snatches you away like a feather torn from the winged messenger. Barbarian! Have you no pity, at least for the small pink flowers, the hollyhocks on Prince Labounoff's azure jacket? Ah, your love, your pitiful love of last year! The pillow on which you dozed, filled with flowers and music; your illusion, your faith—poor you and your pitiful love! Think of the gala of the Duke of B——, think of the terrace, the gallery, the murmur of the fountain! Alas! the beatific smile, the red face and the arrogant paunch of the spirited, artless, wily, deceived Muscovite!

"'Vagabond of sunless days, adventurer of moonless nights!

You will not see again the mutilated Venus of the garden, nor the rickety steps of the entrance; you will not hear again the bird-sound of oars, nor the racing of whistler rats, old rats that shared your insomnia, nor the creaking of the weather vane, now so far away, on the roof, weighed down by old skies, of the Mérone house! All of these things are far away, so far away that they no longer exist, they have never existed, the Past no longer remembers them . . . Look, search and be astonished, tremble . . . You yourself, you have no more past; you have murdered your love, wasted the singing gold of your soul, rudely repudiated your unique faith, obliterated your supreme reality, crushed under your heel the soft grain of wheat that is your heart.

" 'Thunder has struck the oasis; a single tree remains standing in the middle of the desert. The old tree of your solitude will bear no more fruit; the south wind has blown, the dates are rotten at the heart. Die, open yourself to the vermin, become pale as water, then fall and crumble in the wind, old desert tree without fruit or birds, without palm or bark, without breeze or dew! Alone, forever alone in the middle of the desert!'

"Those were my reflections, monsieur le chevalier, those were my cries of regret. My confidences lack a sense of moderation, my confessions lack propriety; do not look at me, do not question me, do not condemn me; I am ashamed, I blush from the depths of my old heart. Pardon me, or, if you feel that I am unworthy of your indulgence, at least pardon love, life, the eternal deep sympathy that weeps and sings at the heart of all things!

"My blood and heart and soul no longer belonged to me. I rejected the idea of separating, even in thought, my destiny from that of la Mérone. Away from my enchantress, I began to doubt the reality of things as well as my own actual existence. Gasping with a nameless anguish, I descended to the street; seriously believing that I had become invisible, I spoke to strangers; their replies surprised, even frightened, me. I touched all the objects that I saw and was astounded that I could still feel and that I was matter, for in la Sulmerre's absence I could not conceive of a reason, or even the semblance of a reason, for my being. I could not admit that my flesh, permeated with love, could be conscious of anything but my lover. A day—what am I saying!—an hour of separation was sufficient to cast me into a state of indescribable collapse, into a void where only my desire and my expectation survived. The premonition of again seeing my beloved quickened in my heart the secret movement of life: her approach, the rustling of her dress, the magic timber of her voice made me start, falter, quake; her embrace filled me with an immense joy, divine and ever new. La Mérone was far from me just a breath ago, and now she is here, at my knees? She, great gods, she herself? And it is not a dream! She, my impossible love, in flesh and bones, in laughter and kisses! I came back to life, shrieking at the miracle. Now misfortune, pain, death itself were banished forever from my destiny. I threw myself at the feet of my goddess, I sobbed in her lap; she had been lost and was now found again, the prodigal little girl of every day, every moment; my soul had no other desire than to celebrate the quotidian festival of seeing her again with a joy that never changed. Judge, monsieur le chevalier, the depth of my passion! And yet all of this fine madness was powerless to allay, in my miserable heart, the suffering caused by the barbs of jealousy or the gnawing of pride, vanity, avarice, and fear. My love was a furious combat of contradictory faults, irreconcilable desires, and opposing vices. My desire to rebel was equaled only by my need to love with no limits, and my thirst for love by my preoccupation with escape; I no longer knew where to turn for wise counsel or from what horizon blew the wind of my madness.

"Nevertheless, months of relentless battle ended with the triumph of sentiment over what remained of my reason, teaching me at the same time that its victories do not diminish, but instead ennoble and enlarge, the vanquished. I conquered, I pacified the realm of my mind. What had been until then but a flame in my heart became a clarity of mind as well. I applied myself with passion to the study of geometry. (Frivolous chevalier, is that really so amusing?) Yes, I returned joyfully to the dear mathematical sciences I had neglected for so long. I recognized in my logical power the awareness of my feelings. The amorous harmony of human understanding intoxicated me: it is all numbers, all cadence; the reality of things and of words is in the rhythm; the entire universe is a boundless song of love. How many qualities we have yet to discover, to conquer, to comprehend in ourselves! Everything is offered to us in our feelings: all that is new, all forms of progress have been there forever. I began to cherish my mind with a father's love. Contemporary of the beginning of things, eternal historiographer of the creative sentiment, I made my mind dance, I made it jump like a little girl. I took pity on it; I taught it love, I taught it to think soundly, to speak truly. All too often human mercy is merely a disguise for contempt, but our forgiving contempt of the rational part of the being is a source of holy and genuine charity. For it is with the bitter love of reason that divine love of the enemy begins in this world, and the end result of every judgment is blind adoration. Whoever you may be, you are at the same time all the wealth and all the poverty of the earth, all love which forgives and all understanding which craves forgiveness. The drama of Paradise lost has been unfolding for years in your anxious breast; the awareness of love ceaselessly usurps the rights of love itself; and from that which is God in you, you draw the conclusion of the divinity of your thinking being, so that the torment created in your heart by Adam's lie cries out for heaven's fire to strike the monstrous tree of science, a tree henceforth sterile but whose flesh without bark threatens you still with the three great bloody nails of the night of Redemption.

"The forgiving love of my miserable reason had the effect of mitigating, to some extent, the sympathetic disgust that the sight of poverty and ugliness always inspired in me. 'The Lord is gracious and full of compassion.' I am not one of those who sells the perfumed oil of his beloved in order to distribute the profits among street-corner beggars. I am not a measure for sentiment; I leave the calculations of charity to the Iscariots. My love of the poor is not a mask for my hatred of the rich. And I am suspicious of the merciful of our times: by their nature they tend to be advocates of the guillotine. The harshness of the rich is sometimes ignorance and laziness, but the hatred of the poor is always the result of an erroneous calculation. The rich man's heart is unfeeling, so be it. But the poor man's heart is bad. The poor man is the reason of the world: he is formidable, proud, and blind. He is not the victim of the social lie: he is the very incarnation of great Mendacity, of irreparable infamy. When Truth shall appear, stone in hand, and the teeth of the monster are broken, the poor man will be cured and not avenged. For poverty is an illness, a plague upon the earth, a cancer devouring our heart. Let the rich fornicate until dawn in the festive hall, I will not crawl under the table to lick the wounds of Lazarus. Lazarus will use the sword and be master tomorrow; and he will have his prostitutes and his poor. I question revolutions, sterile anticipators of the revelation. The heart of Truth is not the heart of a creature, glistening and fragile; love is not the favor of a lost woman. The heart of Truth is a stone in a torrent, drunk with purity, turbulence, and light; and Love is the terrible master of the new Jerusalem. Man has come, but very little has come of Man. Man will soon return in his true form, which is that of the master of the new Jerusalem. And it will be—believe me, chevalier—a matter of much less than an instant of our earthly life.

"I went toward the poor. They welcomed my sincerity with distrust, I learned their secret with no surprise. How many of my own characteristics I recognized in them! There is scarcely anything surprising in the passage from a world where one does not think what one says to a world where one cannot say what one thinks. I sat down at the laborer's table, I leaned over the pallet of the dying man, I cast food into the horrible maw of hunger. And I shook with disgust at the sight of the infamous tears of gratitude. One day a very old and infirm soldier threw himself at my feet, calling me his savior. My heart overflowed with a frightful commotion. 'Put him to the sword, the sword! Finish him off! You will give alms when your love learns how to multiply loaves of bread. Today you must kill, you must kill!'

"Despite my care in keeping these charitable debaucheries secret, Clarice knew of them. Her natural goodness, like that of a sensual child, at once became enamored of this inferior ideal. There was much of a boy—and a charming boy—in her. She wished to follow me on my pilgrimages to garrets, and it was with great difficulty that I dissuaded her. It is too early in the day of time for the betrothal of love and pity. More sun is required, a great noontime of love, to make of the bitter little root of our pity something illuminated with flowers and intoxicating to bees. Man, Man is approaching! He walks on the sea, followed by a holy procession of mountains smitten with love. He is handsome, powerful, terrible: the first stone of Jerusalem gleams in his hand; he kisses the blood-soaked face of the defeated, dying monster. All human flesh is aflame with immense, joyful pity! For it is immense and joyful, the pity which runs to meet strength and beauty!

"When Annalena became irritated by my refusals, I responded with a small hypocritical smile, 'Patience, my dear child, patience. There is no hurry, to tell the truth. I am still so far from knowing the real poor!' It was neither a bad or a false reason even though I had another, better and more unusual, that I hid jealously. When one has two explanations of something, it is prudent to keep the simpler one to oneself; for the less clear reason often is more successful in convincing an uninitiated spirit, by which I mean still naively in love with profound pathetic thoughts. The second mysterious reason is this: nothing diminishes us as much in the eyes of our fellow man as our pity for an incurable evil. Charity will seem beautiful to creatures of love when it shall be able to return sight to the blind, hearing to the deaf, movement to the paralyzed, and life to the dead. Louis le Grand barred the door of Versailles to those wounded in his wars. The heart of the king knew the heart of man.

"My capricious charity had two companions: the melancholy of evening and the elation of morning. The first usually was trailed through unhealthy, nauseating alleys by the mangy, obscene, and starving spirit of my faithful friend the dog; the other by a puny philosopher banished from France, quite old and of a disquieting appearance, whom the innkeepers of the port and the managers of houses of ill repute saluted reverently by the name of vicomte de Flagny. This M. de Flagny belonged to the category of men whom one dreams about all of one's life after seeing them only once, remembering the person but not the time or place of meeting. He had the head of a jovial toad above the body of a suspicious grasshopper, grimy trappings, and the habit of speaking about the temple of Solomon while fondling matrons, young girls, and little girls. I saw him two or three times a week at the nighttime sessions of one of those supposedly secret brotherhoods which at that time proliferated all through the Veneto, with no other apparent object than to bring together men of widely differing birth and conviction but dedicated to the same bizarre cult of mystery and instability. Wine and eloquence flowed like water; here the pitcher is emptied and the church stumbles; there the glasses are refilled and the temple grows larger before one's eyes. The German prince hobnobs with the author of a famous lampoon; the monk converses in hushed tones with the clairvoyant; the member from Geneva appears: the master's brow darkens. The intemperate

Flagny mumbles, between two bottles of wine, the 149th psalm:

> Let the high praises of God be in their mouth, and a
> two-edged sword in their hand;
> To execute vengeance upon the heathen, and pun-
> ishments upon the people;
> To bind their kings with chains, and their nobles with
> fetters of iron;
> To execute upon them the judgment written: this
> honor have all his saints.

"How much childishness is apparent in the affairs of man to him who understands truly the spirit of associations of this genre! How you would have laughed at the silly speech of welcome that I intoned in a voice of flame and wind above the hundred perukes of a dumbfounded and charmed assembly. Love is so high, so deep, so pure, so incredible! No matter if you make it say or do this or that; its spirit embraces everything, its shoulders are powerful; have no fear of adding a little loving foolishness to the burden of infamy that the god carries so lightly. German prince, author of satires, monk, seer—all are moved, exclaim, leap to their feet, come running; I am applauded, flattered, jostled, deafened; disturbing cries break out on all sides: 'The Initiate, the Herald, the second Baptist! the new Bethabara before celestial Jerusalem!' The door resounded with three furious blows: silence. Surprise and terror were limned on all faces . . . Well then! would it not be in fact the member from Geneva? The master's brow recovered its serenity . . .

"Ordinarily M. de Flagny followed my love gallops at the

little trot of his hobby-horse of fraternity. From time to time I stopped to wait for him; after an instant that seemed eternal, and with the most innocent and most satisfied air in the world, he would catch up with me, and I welcomed him with a tremendous volley of derision and malediction. Although the good fellow lacked neither spirit or heart, he remained attached to the entrails of his motherland by an invisible cord; his view ended fatuously at the wall of the horizon and, even though he spoke often of nature with tears in his eyes and his voice, I was never taken in; and that was because I felt that he gave that sacred name not to love, principle of things, but to a combination of forces and laws, to an assemblage of specific universes, to an immensity formed of precise little corners hospitable to weights and measures. I sweated blood and water to make him see reason, to make him know that there is no reality apart from love, which is holy Spirit or Spirit of truth, that is to say, adoration of God for himself through man; that in this holy Trinity all wisdom resides; that, finally, knowledge is the relationship of things and not things in themselves. The excellent fellow would not rest until he fell again into the common error of philosophers of nature. Confusing the principle of things with the sequence of the laws to which they are subject, he drew from the concept of nature that of the 'natural,' unconsciously played on the two words, made of nature a 'natural' thing, created a supreme law of the absolute necessity of laws, and inevitably concluded with the old idea of falseness and truth, without realizing that what appears false insofar as it is contrary to the law imposed on reason can very well be true in the eyes of the principle revealed to sentiment.

"The abuse of great words and of old smoky wines sometimes caused eloquence to swell into vehemence and contro-
versy to degenerate into dispute; the brotherhood of mystical
old fools then divided itself into two enemy camps, next separated into small incoherent groups, and finally disintegrated into
Bacchic, irreconcilable personalities. Then, when the assembly
found itself divided into as many opinions as there were heads,
one of these weird fellows ran to open wide the doors of an
adjacent salon, and a lively crowd of beauties from all over the
world came running to mingle their gay warblings with the dull
and angry noise of a hundred extravagant monologues.

"That was the usual signal for me to leave, for now that my
old roué's heart had tasted true love, the spectacle of orgy had
nothing to offer me that did not revolt my spirit and my senses.
Nothing is as odious to true affection as the simulation of passion and the false semblance of joy, and I know of nothing closer
to pain than pleasure which leaves the soul indifferent. Despite
the sympathy, even the admiration, which the viscount had felt
for my enchantress the first time he saw her, sometimes he tried
to detain me amidst the wicked company by mocking my ex-
clusive passion, like that of a virtuous young bridegroom; but
my invariable reply to these pranks was to speak in praise of love,
of the great solitary love which finds its happiness not in the fidelity of its subject, but in the simple respect of itself. And all
the while that I made the man's head spin with a thousand more
or less contradictory arguments, I was pushing him gently toward the door leading to the street, and there I cast him out,
stunned and shivering, into the great silence of the dawn, the
large empty silence, pale and unaware of the new day.

"I can think of nothing more deliciously distressing than an aimless stroll through the poor sections of a great city, particularly after a night spent in discriminating, costly debauchery. Even in my first youth I pursued with passion this morose pleasure, so rich in devastating contrasts. Consequently, there does not exist a blind alley so obscure anywhere in Europe, from Whitechapel in London to Freta in Warsaw, that I do not know better than the world of my own heart, so full of bitterness and gloom. I am the friend of hypocritical old windows, the confidant of hostile barred doors, the accomplice of cellars where someone once descended and never came back up . . . My memory is a strange city where the rue du Chant-des-Oiseaux in Frankfurt leads to Soho and to Mile End Road by way of the low roads of Kiev and the Ghetto of Venice. And my soul is a church, Saint-Clément Danes, sooty and slimy in the midst of a hideous tangle of villainous alleys in Hamburg or Naples. I know which stones of Fleet Street shook under the vagabond footsteps of Samuel Johnson, which windows of the Ile Saint-Louis watched the comings and goings of Restif★ and of Jean-Jacques,★ which panes of glass of the Avenue des Tilleuls rang under Gluck's fingers. My heart has an affinity for dull, mute, inanimate things, and a secret instinct guides my feverish old legs toward desolate places where some monstrous sorrow still hopes for redemption. Let the misty light of an East End tavern attract my attention and at once a strange voice whispers in my ear, 'Enter, this is where you might encounter your lost soul.' I notice an angle in the wall, moss-covered and smelling of urine, a broken, rusted gutter, a mound of refuse or some other charming object of that sort; I stop, I dally there dreaming of some past mistress, ugly and vicious; I regret someone who has died and whom I never loved; I recall distant, empty moments which I care about as I do about myself . . . I do not know what sullen toad, fattened on filth and bitterness, croaks day and night in me, half-crushed beneath the heavy, icy stone of my heart.

"If only I could open up my old skull, pointed and plucked under its peruke, like a box of surprises, in order to show you the image of people and things that memory retraces there and that no words could describe! You would recognize the friend who speaks to you now, with the long legs of a hanged man and the same wrinkled, sharp face, but ten years younger; and by his side you could see, hopping, gesticulating, and blowing into a red and yellow handkerchief, a small old man shivering in a green suit too long and too big, a snake shedding its skin, a frozen nut in too large a shell; and you would see a powdered macaque tail dancing on the old man's nape, and a long épée hanging crookedly on his cicadalike derrière. And the hesitant step of the two noblemen would surprise you, as would the dirty color of the hour and of the water, the flaking walls of the houses, and the supernatural silence of the sky. And you would follow the maddest of Brettinoros and the most scatterbrained Flagny through the *calli*★ and the *campielli*★ unknown to people of means, and up worm-eaten staircases hostile to their inebriated footsteps, and into hovels of which the sight alone would nauseate you. And there, in the presence of pallets full of vermin and children, by greasy tables where young couples withered by misery dip their dry crusts in transparent gruel, you would find an excellent occasion to rid yourself of both your useless old tears and of your offensive and horrible gold.

"The amiable Flagny made his offering serenely, as a man of property convinced of the usefulness of alms; as for myself, I had a more savage and more tortured way of helping my fellow man. The viscount had only to obey his natural goodness; his task was easy. Myself, I repressed the surge of my love, and my distress was profound. My silence was a reproach to the poor for their ugliness, their bitterness, their resignation. Nor could I forgive them for my powerlessness to ameliorate their lot. Alas! the blind leading the blind, the poor helping the poor! From the attic window I contemplated the glory of the ocean horizons; my life opened all its doors to eternity's breath, and I marveled that things so beautiful, so great, and so holy could pardon the frailty and the stunted ugliness of my charity. 'These are the alms of evil love,' I repeated to myself endlessly, 'This is the compassion of failed love, of a love that lies, lies to its own immortality, that proclaims itself ephemeral and useless, and that allows itself to be convinced by its own lie to the point where it declines, grows old, and dies. What are we waiting for that is not already there in our awestruck eyes, in our intoxicated hearts? Is not today composed of all our yesterdays, all our tomorrows? Is not eternity instantaneous? On your feet, on your feet! Abandon yourself to your love! Call upon the blind, the deaf, the paralyzed to rise, to rise and walk upon the sea! For if that is your love of a living creature, how impoverished must be the heart of those who bury their dead!' Overcome with disgust, hatred, and pity, I threw my purse to the gravediggers so that they might sing my praises while inhaling the corrupt wine of life.

"The 'object' of a love, particularly of a very deep love, can never be its 'end.' In the case of great adoration, the creature is never more than a medium. Authentic love hungers for reality, and the only reality is in God. If grand passion usually founders in disenchantment and despair, it is never only in the earthly sense of those words, because in ascending to the adoration of the Impersonal, of the gentle, all-powerful Love our father, its loss is repaid a hundred times over. Profound love is a painful uplifting to the delightful dwelling place of chastity, simplicity, and childhood. Disillusionment causes us to lose the world and gain Him whose realm is not of this world. The dawning of faith, charity, and of infinite sympathy for man in my heart made me clearly understand that the role played by la Sulmerre in the drama of my life was drawing to its close. What I loved in Annalena was that which no one else but me could know, that which no one could steal from me, that which no doubt even she had never discovered. And yet, as the lover of a woman, I suffered every imaginable torment, for I felt my fear of imaginary danger grow worse hour by hour with a thousand well-founded suspicions. The accursed circle of Don Juans drew constantly tighter around my beautiful one, who became more receptive and more flirtatious every day; and there was not one among these odious roués of her entourage who did not delude himself with the sweet hope of seeing his ardor rewarded at the first opportunity.

"My patience was at an end: the impertinence of these callow youths had now passed all bounds, and their persistence in staring at me expressed only too eloquently how little importance they attached to my ready triumph and to the ephemeral faithfulness of my beloved. As for Labounoff, after our chance encounter in Calle Selle Rampani, never did he show the slightest resentment toward me for having supplanted him, for which I often reproached myself as a lapse in the obligations of friendship. At first I did not know how to take the prince's conduct. The contrast between his passionate confidence and the indifferent attitude which I noticed in him continued to surprise me; nevertheless it was clear that the crafty boyar, expert as he was in matters of gallantry, had not been slow to understand la Mérone's nature. Being very little concerned, therefore, about obtaining anything other than what this type of woman usually granted her lovers, he desired only to be my immediate successor in the good graces of the fickle lady; and his patient, wise jealousy was directed entirely against a certain Baron Zegollary, who seemed willing to contest his rank among those aspiring to the favors of the lovable Mérone.

"This Zegollary was certainly the ugliest and most repulsive being in the world. I do not believe that I have ever met in my life a meaner, more narrow-minded or vainer character. Despite his age, which was well past sixty, and the grotesque protuberances conferred upon his body by the bizarre aggregation of a large livid goiter, a heavy, quivering stomach, and an enormous pair of buttocks, eternally in motion, the hideous braggart stubbornly insisted on blindly mimicking the airs and graces of fashionable young men and the affectations of the libertines whom he ordinarily frequented; for, bleary-eyed and suffering from gout as he was, the boor thought it amusing to crown his innumerable Hungarian absurdities with the sin of the Bulgarians. In spite of my distaste, I could only laugh at the killing looks with which la Sulmerre honored this noxious flower, who stuck to her more closely than anyone, and each day I was astonished that Labounoff could take offense at it. However, the prince's suspicions about my mistress were only too well-founded, and from that time on I had numerous occasions to notice that the Muscovite had every right to pride himself on understanding the heart of beautiful women, or rather, as he used to say, 'the essential organ of these dear little doves of wenches.' "

At this point M. de Pinamonte, interrupting his narrative and fishing from the recesses of his diabolical soutane an ancient snuffbox from the blessed past, sneezed more than ten times into his beautiful Armenian handkerchief and, all crimson from a most clumsily feigned coughing fit, rubbed his poor serpent's eyes furiously and at length, much ashamed to be seen brimming with old tears of regret and of love.

"Ah, chevalier of my heart! friend of chance and of the devil! It is surely not possible that you too have never known the venomous sweetness of some tender dove of a wench. I know . . . no, I do not know your life . . . ; but from the first moment, your eloquent eyes revealed everything to me, last night on the Ponte Tappio. The tender passion of a hussy, the maternal sweetness in the frenzy of vice, the artless friendship of a sister in the heart of Messalina, the rudeness of insult and the weakness of compassion, pity and the distaste for pity, the jealousy one savors like an old Cyprus wine mixed with bitter aphrodisiacs; all of these horrible and delicious things are contained in the magic name of Annalena-Clarice de Mérone, false countess of Sulmerre, the temperamental adventuress, formidable and gentle, maternal and nymphomaniacal. Sweet—oh, yes, by God! and how sweet—for she had given me violent nights and tender days. There was child and she-goat in her flesh, and in her soul both angel and baboon. Her spirit was rare and charming, her heart . . . but a love like mine has no need of excuses.

"All that remains, monsieur le chevalier, is for me to describe to you in a few words the inevitable betrayal which caused the abrupt rupture of our relations. The scene seems to me too licentious for me to feel free to linger over it. Should you be desirous, however, of knowing the intimate details of that priceless spectacle I had the ghastly pleasure and the laughable misfortune to witness, a few confidential sketches drawn from memory would be more than sufficient, I believe, to satisfy your curiosity.

"One night, when according to Scythian custom, he had drunk wine to the point of indiscretion, Prince Serge, leading me into a remote gallery of the palace of B———, bellowed in my ear between two unctuous, grumbling kisses, 'By Hercules and Labounoff! Little pigeon of a count, little soul of a duke, soon you will no longer have anything, by my faith, with which to reproach yourself. Word has reached me that you are leaving Venice this very night for some business which cannot wait. Know then that my preparations are as thorough as yours and that soon my dearest wish will be granted, at your expense, of course, cuckold of the devil that you are! By Hercules! never have I been in a better humor! What an obscene and exquisite whim of our charming minx. From now on, no more competitiveness between us; it is only fair to allow us to finally enjoy, in peace, a common bliss.'

"Although dead drunk, the tormentor did not fail to note the effect of his strange remarks on the spirit of his victim.

Apparently the fumes of his wine were not enough to hide the fire of indignation and shame on my brow. In spite of the efforts he made to change his tone and turn the thing into a joke, I found it hard to enter into his game, particularly since his allusion to my voyage gave plausibility to the vile conspiracy, for in fact a most urgent affair summoned me to Livorno. I judged it not at all opportune to listen to the continuation of this singular oration. The insult had cut me to the quick. Distress overcoming resolution, I deferred my departure and determined to break with the ungrateful woman within the hour.

"Followed by the fatherly Giovanni, I ran to the abode of my mistress; but the strumpet, who had not ceased to complain of vapors since the sun rose, had already left both her bed and her house without the knowledge of her maids. Nothing more was needed to cause me to lose the little calm that remained to me after the prince's confidences. Nevertheless, the ingenious Giovanni soon laid his plans and sent out a legion of emissaries. Ironic Phoebe★ assisted our designs, and the corruptibility of gondoliers was of some help to us as well; thus, after an hour of beating our way across the city, we were ready, Giovanni and I, to march against the enemy.

"I shall not go into detail concerning this farcical expedition; I have no recollection of it. My head down, I ran like a lost soul this way and that, tripping over the rubble of my ruined life with each step. Crossing the sinister Campiello del Piovan; an old house situated in a most villainous quarter; a foul-smelling, greasy staircase strewn with orange peels; finally, a great blow of Giovanni's épée against the door: these are the only things I remember. I regained some control over my senses only at the instant when the door was opened to us. I caught a glimpse of Labounoff naked as a hand. At the sight of me, he backed up a few steps. I entered.

"By the flickering light of a single candle, I saw Clarice-Annalena Mérone, countess of Sulmerre, disrobed in the Arcadian style and lounging on the most voluptuous of couches: her brother Alessandro was her featherbed, Zegollary her bolster, and milord Edward Gordon Colham a pretty bauble for her charming little fingers to idle with. Life very nearly deserted me.

"My first movement was to grasp my faithful épée; my second was to smile as I recalled that I was Brettinoro, Benedetto, and Guidoguerra; and finally, by the trick of a bizarre association, my mind seized on the image of the abbé de Rancé;★ and this subtle and preposterous connection succeeded in lifting my spirits.

"None of the contorted nudes of the drunken mythological group was stained with the blood of vengeance. No one died that night; no, to tell the truth, no one. For my youth and my illusions were already dead, by the fork and tail of the devil! dead and buried for many long years.

"Sometimes a violent surprise clarifies the real nature of our feelings with a certainty that we would wait for in vain from a mind continually troubled by excessive preoccupations. Thus, confronted by the ignoble and seductive spectacle that I watched in fascination, I recognized belatedly that I had been cruelly mocked in every way by my depraved imagination. The destiny of melancholy buffoons of my type is to pursue all through their lives some fruitless phantom of passion, art, or philosophy, then to find rest in the holy and unique reality of God's bosom.

"After the first rush of emotion, I made my excuses to the sheepish lovers for the sudden interruption of their frolics; and, while joking pleasantly about the youthful ardor of their transports, I complimented them on the Attic grace of their games and implored them to return to their unfinished masterpiece. Labounoff at once gave the signal for a new assault. Just gods! but the prince had done well! Without any difficulty, I confess that for a moment I felt a strong desire to participate in that agreeable combat. It would have taken very little for me to throw myself into the amorous melee; however, such was the violence of my belligerent envy that the mere sight of arms and wounds was enough to appease it. All the while that her friends offered her their delicate attentions, my dear Mérone amused herself with sending me mischievous kisses full of tenderness; never had the little imp seemed so beautiful, nor so graciously adorned with all the attractions of innocence. The chance circumstance of licentious poses took nothing away from the instinctive modesty of her bearing; at last I saw her as nature had created her; I no longer doubted the artlessness of her loves. The spectacle ravished me with joy. In particular, I was deeply touched by the expressions of affection lavished on his sister by young Alessandro; nevertheless, while heaping praise on the principal actors in this scene, I could not fail to register admiration for the secondary roles; for there was not one, including even that bulbous, blighted Zegollary, who did not demonstrate on this occasion a competence and a dexterity worthy of the greatest acclaim. As far as my dear mistress was concerned, no sooner was the harmless scuffle over than I pressed her tenderly against my breast and placed a couple of fraternal kisses on her brow, which was again reddening. Why, chevalier, do we not break the stupid habit of considering as our fellow creature an Eve whose spirit and flesh we will never know? For how can we understand a being who is able to be completely faithful to us in the same instant that she is taking the fire of an entire troop of guards?

"Feeling that I was cured forever of my former foolishness, I gaily took leave of my friends without for a moment dreaming of reproaching them for their remarkable behavior toward me. I hurried to my banker. Nothing in my estimation equals in nobility the fine head of a treacherous rogue engraved in palpable, melodious gold. I made my farewells first to the dens and bawdy houses of Venice in the company of the gentle, innocent viscount, and then to the city itself. My foolish friendship for Edward Gordon Colham was of brief duration. I discovered in milord a spirit already too much influenced by the dangerous frequentation of women.

"On the day fixed for departure, I paid my last visit to the sweet mistress of my life. I briskly crossed the dark galleries and silent rooms. Without knocking, I entered the salon of the spinet. My ravishing one was there, paler than usual, sadly lurking in the little corner so dear to my former reveries, between the fireplace and the oak chest, under the Hogarth and in front of the Longhi. 'The hour has come, my dear Annalena,' I say to her simply. 'Alas, monsieur,' she replies with the voice of a child, 'Why must you be so little in tune with the age? Hate me, but do not despise me; for it is certain that I will be forgiven much, very much.' I could not help but smile at this bizarre application of my past sermons. Nonetheless, in looking into the eyes of my beauty, I read there the same response as in the fine gaze of an innocent young dog, warm and faithful. 'Ah! why have I not told you before this the unfortunate story of my life!' she continued. 'I have never known a father; my mother was a . . .' I put my hand over her lips. 'Too late, too late, my dear child!' Filial tears ran down her poor, sweet cheeks. She rose as if to go to the spinet. I guessed her intention and stopped her in the middle of the chamber. Ah, poor love; ah, sad truth! My glance in the tall mirror met my glance. My old age was apparent for the first time in all its candor. 'The time for little love affairs is past,' I tell myself, 'It grows late in the day of the world; love is near.' Then, turning toward my lovely one, 'The moment, in its turn, has come, my adored Clarice.' I took several steps toward the door. La Sulmerre did not waver. La Sulmerre remained as if rooted to the spot. Two very old and very silly verses sang in my memory:

> *Though Lot's wife was turned to salt,*
> *She menstruated, a woman's fault.*

"I released the door lock. I began to open the door. The cry of a gondolier sounded in the distance. Then everything fell silent again.

"Numb to the point of feeling no surprise at the sudden calming of a soul which had known so many alarms, I began to walk in the direction of Calle Barozzi. There I found my baggage already outside and, as on so many previous occasions, the staircase of my house resounding with the laughter and curses of porters. The good Giovanni was waiting at the door for me in his traveling clothes. Flagny leaned listlessly on his shoulder; lady Gualdrada sobbed into her lap. Although I sincerely loved both the scatterbrained viscount and the unlucky fortune-teller, their pathetic state surprised me. They still feared the hour of parting, and my soul had conquered Him from whom nothing can part us.

"In a soft voice and with a lighthearted gesture, I gave my servant the order to proceed to the landing stage. The porters followed us, humming. Flagny spoke of the future, Gualdrada of the days to come. I smiled at both their comments. The sun, direct satellite of love, breathed its wind of fire and dreams over all of the blazing Molo. I embraced Sciancato's widow; I pressed to my breast the innocent enemy of tyrants. A breeze made of tears and laughter swelled the sails of the impatient three-master. We lifted anchor. The *Riva degli Schiavoni* took wing in the buoyant air. I ran to the stern: on the swift-moving bank Gualdrada waved her handkerchief, Flagny his hat. Not a sigh or a groan escaped me; my heart was already like a ripe fruit in the great silence. Giovanni looked at me with surprise. The Ponte Ca' di Dio faded from my view; the Isola di San Giorgio disappeared in its turn. The air was as pure as the laughter of farewell. With a large sign of the cross I embraced the beauty of my sweet Venice, the melancholy of my past happiness, the life and the death of Annalena the Initiatrix. And my flesh shivered with the voluptuousness of prayer.

"The light of the sky is swift, the mind of man even swifter; but the truth that reveals itself to emotion surpasses the swiftness of both sun and thought. Suddenly I felt alone, alone and face to face with myself. Prayer had wiped from my lips the taste of the worm-eaten fruit of love gathered in an Eden attacked by the plague of Adam. I understood why God no longer wanted, no longer was able, to reveal himself to man; why love between creatures was no longer the presence of the living God. A woman's body is a cross, and a woman's kiss a sponge of vinegar;* the husband is crucified on the wife, the lover on his sweetheart, the mother on the son. Lean over cradles, enter into tombs: falsehood is everywhere. It flickers like the will-o'-the-wisp of marshes on the face of a child, like the light of a sepulchral lamp on the brow of old age. It runs from year to year, from century to century, as the viscous sediment of the sea dances from wave to wave. Your father betrayed you, as did your mother, and your friend, and she in whom you believed you had found your heart's peace. Houses look at each other with mistrust; however, less falsehood is concealed in a wall built in front of a wall than in the look a woman raises to her lover's eyes. Beware of your child: the dream of his nights is full of hate, and he dares not laugh or cry; the hand of terrible silence is over his mouth. Falsehood, cold calculation, the heart's insensitivity spy on you from their hiding places. What your mother loves in you is not you; what your beloved adores in you belongs to someone else, to everyone else; and each is betrayed in the name of all until each has learned to deceive himself. The sun will dry out your skin, the moon will whiten your hair, and you will be like a dead tree in the wind and like the leaf blown toward the sea; and when the hour strikes you will still say, 'Where then is the word of truth?' And he who has not suffered from his love and who has accepted his love just as he found it, that person has never loved, and his heart rots in falsehood like the worm's carcass in the rotted fruit. But he who has suffered from his love for a person and in repudiating that love has returned to the eternally pure source of a contaminated river, that person knows Love from the beginning of time, that person walks in the effulgence of God's presence.

"Anyone but you, chevalier, would have interrupted me more than once in the course of my overly long tale, to set against my idea of unique and therefore divine love the multiplicity of sentiments that govern the world, and thus to call my attention to the small number of relationships which represent the diverse manifestations of human affection. What could be fairer, however, than that the one who assures the propagation of the being flows directly from the principle of the being? If the creature radiant with beauty, truth, and guilelessness is the perceptible manifestation of God's love for Himself, is it not in the sublime attachment to some creature that we would have to look first, in a simpler and purer life, for an expression of our love of the terrible and gentle Father of things? And what does it matter that this attachment, even when it is deep and sincere, does not last as long as life, if it causes the mortal heart to beat with the rhythm of the Love without end! Every affection is composed of a dream and a reality: the dream is on earth, whose days are numbered; reality is in the Eternal. Life according to the world is the shadow of a mist, a feeling of doubt in the nocturnal dream of a madman; but the feeblest desire of true love already contains all the reality of Heaven, and all will be pardoned to the creature who loved with a supreme love after having long burned with the worst. Moreover, is not the folly of lovers the first mystical ring linking the entire harmonious chain of conservative feelings to God's bosom, from the mother's affection to the tenderheartedness of a man for a stone in the street? Would my agonizing appeal to a life not poisoned at its source then be such an insane thing? In a word, is it not he who has tasted the most sullied love whose lips will be refreshed in the brightness of the most limpid?

"We set sail toward Manfredonia,* once unconcerned with joy and grief. Following the flight of birds and the passage of clouds with my gaze, I reviewed in my mind both the history of my own affection and the principal episodes of the intrigues in which I was involved. I cast about vainly in my memory for the example of a single love of which one could say, 'That one was both deep and happy.' I evoked grand passions, those which break ties and overcome obstacles, and they appeared to me wearing the hideous features of betrayal, lassitude, contempt, and disgust. I examined solemn, calm love, the great procreator nourished on the respect of tradition and the future; and I trembled at the sight of so much mediocrity, resignation, and boredom. Finally, I cried out for the love of man; and my fellow man came to lie at my feet, miserable, suspicious, bound in chains and dying of hunger. Then I raised my hands to the sky, saying, 'May you be blessed, O Love, O Our Father of the earthly Paradise lost! O You, all that has been, O You, all that which will be, even to the temporal sojourn, and is no more! Abandoned by Adam, victim of the Pharisee! O pure treasure of those who have lost everything! How just it is that I can know you only from the dark depth of the abyss of grief! How beautiful is your law of expiation! And what sweetness in this bleak anticipation of your last incarnation, O Holy Spirit, O Spirit of Truth, O Paraclete!' "*

The noble Antisthène was silent. I looked up. The holy man sniffled hideously into his beautiful Armenian handkerchief.

"Such is," he added, wiping his eyes, "such is, dear confidant of my heart, the edifying and very simple story of Manto the tender, the faithless, and the dead. Not the dead lady of Vercelli, monsieur le Benjamin, but well and truly dead, soul and flesh. Yes, agreeable monsieur; our lady of Sulmerre is no longer of this world. Two anonymous messages arrived in quick succession last year to inform me of illness and of death. You would not believe how much I was grieved by these tidings."

At the garden gate I turned for the customary final bow. I saw M. de Pinamonte bareheaded, in the melting glory of the setting sun. Two heavy tears trickled down his mirthful face. He stooped as if to pick up something at his feet. His poor trembling hands lifted up, with some effort, a large stone hidden among the weeds.

"May this soul, so sweet and so humble, be the witness of our farewells," he intoned in a grave voice. And he added, "The Absurd, the famous absurd alone remains to us. Whoever has ears understands!"

"*A bientôt,* monsieur," I called to him from the street corner.

Nothing was less simple than to discern the true and the false, the sincere and the feigned, in the story of Antisthène. Only the unbearable scene of the betrayal seemed to me, if not entirely imagined, at the very least exaggerated beyond the limits

---

179

of plausibility. Over the following two days I amused myself by putting down on paper all sorts of reflections on the subject of my eccentric, but on the third day I destroyed my scribblings and threw them in the fire; for I discovered no more than a bizarre tangle of contradictory judgments and of maxims that made no sense. Whatever I did, however, I could not refrain from evoking a hundred times a day the disturbing person of my hollow dream; and even though my feelings for him were composed as much of scorn as of admiration, I passed a fort-night scouring the streets of Naples in the hope of coming across, or at least recognizing, the way to his residence. Fortunately, I was left with a vivid memory of the house and its street, for I was never able to find either one or the other except in my mind. I had no better luck in my quest for information. Those who were best informed sent me to the works of Machiavelli or of Alighieri; others, more expeditious in these matters because they were less erudite, quite simply sent me to the devil; and, despite all the mysticism of his Pinamonte, the unfortunate Benjamin found more perceptiveness among the ignorant than among the scholarly.

Toward the middle of October I received from Copenhagen orders to proceed with all possible haste to Saxony, where my brother the plenipotentiary had been expecting me for two months. The matter did not permit delay. The wording of the note made me fear that the King and the Council were at the end of their patience. I dispatched my affairs and climbed into my carriage with the sentiment of once again being separated from la Mérone, once again and for all time.

At the moment we turned the corner of the street, a curse

from the postillion, a great brouhaha of laughter, and the howling of a wounded animal made me look out. On the muddy pavement lay an amorphous mass of blood, brains, and hair, which some grimy street urchins were amusing themselves by crushing under their bare heels. "It's nothing, my lord," one of them called to me laughing, "only the mangy old dog from the Ponte Tappio which your horses have just reduced to a pulp." A stroke of the whip dispersed the rabble and we continued on our way.

The End

Endnotes

pp. 7, 37, 64, 120, 129. Poniatowski. Stanislas II [1732–1798], the last king of Poland [1764–1795].

p. 7, et seq. Antisthène. Appears to be the author's coinage, a composite of *anti* and *sthenia,* denoting vigor or force. [Gk. *sthenos,* strength].

p. 15. Frère Albéric. There were various poets named Albéric; the two most likely possibilities in this context would seem to be Albéric, the second abbot of Citeaux [1109], who initiated the Cistercian reform, or, more likely, Alberico da Montecassino [1101–1146], who as a child had a vision of a voyage through Inferno, Purgatory, and Paradise guided by Saint Peter and two angels. He became a monk, and in collaboration with Pietro Diacono, wrote of his vision, considered to be one of the sources of Dante's *Divine Comedy.*

p. 18. *rii.* In Venetian dialect, the singular is *rio.*

pp. 22, 92, 105. Saana. Appears to be a mythical, primitive land, but could be a variant on Sana, capital of Yemen, a city with a long and turbulent history, variously spelled San'a or Sanaa when transliterated from the Arabic. Its location in the ancient world is appropriate in context.

p. 29. Sémiramis of the North. Sémiramis, a Babylonian or Assyrian queen who became a legendary heroine. Designation for Catherine the Great of Russia.

p. 30. Manto. One of the names of Clarice-Annalena de Sulmerre. Manto, daughter of Tiresias, soothsayer of Thebes, was sometimes called the moon goddess.

Cynthie. Cynthia, from *Cynthus,* mountain on Delos where she was born, another name for Artemis.

Undines. Water nymphs.

p. 35. Callirhoë. Variously spelled Callirhoé, Callirrhoë, Kallirhoé. Daughter of the river god Achelous. Name commonly used for various mythological women.

According to one legend, she was the object of hopeless love of a priest of Dionysus.

p. 38. Maritorne. A remarkably ugly serving maid in *Don Quixote*.

p. 39. Atman, or Atma [Sanskrit]. The inner self; divine consciousness residing in the individual; the soul; supreme spirit.

Paracelsus [1493–1541] (pseudonym). Swiss-born alchemist and physician, father of hermetic medicine.

Nettesheim. Heinrich Agrippa de Nettesheim [1486–1535], born in Germany: writer, physician, philosopher, magician, cabalist.

p. 53. Arouet. The family name of Voltaire.

p. 60. jerboa. A nocturnal Old World jumping rodent.

p. 65. Astarte and Amodeus. Astarte or Astaroth, Ashtoreth, Istar: goddess of heaven, protectress. Asmodeus, diabolical personage.

p. 74. introit. An antiphon, verse from a psalm, and the Gloria Patri, sung while the priest approaches the altar to celebrate Mass or Holy Communion; a piece of music sung or played at the beginning of a worship service.

matins. Morning prayers.

p. 79. Allobroge. The Allobroges, a people of Gaul noted for their wealth and also for their quarrelsome nature. The name returned to usage during the time of the Revolution.

p. 82. Riquet à la Houppe. From a folk tale by Charles Perrault [1628–1703], in which Prince Riquet, who is intelligent but ugly, weds a beautiful but stupid princess; thanks to the fairies, his mind and her beauty are exchanged. The moral drawn is that love prevents us from seeing the flaws of those we love and endows them with our own qualities.

p. 85. Enobarbus. Domitius Enobarbus, consul in A.D. 32, first husband of Agrippine and father of Nero. After deserting Antony, his friend, he kills himself.

Sporus. A favorite of Nero.

p. 86. Agnes. Could refer to a naive, innocent character in Molière's *L'Ecole des Femmes;* or to Saint Agnes [early 4th century], a celebrated Roman martyr. According to tradition, she refused marriage, stating that she could have no spouse but Jesus Christ. Her suitors revealed her Christianity, and in punishment she was exposed in a brothel.

Beatrix. A spiritual guide in Dante, who created in her one of the most celebrated women in all of literature. There is also a Beatrix, bestower of blessings, in medieval legend, a nun devoted to the cult of the Virgin Mary. She sinned but repented and was forgiven.

Laurette de Sado. Probably the Laura loved by Petrarch, though his contemporaries believed that the name [from *laurea,* laurelwreath] was chosen to illustrate that the love of woman symbolized the love of glory. Petrarch insisted that his love of Laura was authentic, but there is no documentation of any real Laura, not even the most generally accepted possibility, Laura de Noves, married to Ugo de Sade in 1325.

p. 104. Cythera. Aegean island associated with Aphrodite, where she had a magnificent temple. Perhaps Cytherea, another name for Aphodite, is intended.

p. 106, 176. ". . . a woman's kiss [is] a sponge of vinegar." Allusion to the Roman soldiers who gave the dying Jesus a sponge soaked in vinegar.

p. 121. In describing *Women at the Menagerie,* a painting by Longhi, Milosz refers to the animal portrayed as, variously, a buffalo and a bull. There is a Longhi, however, called *Exhibition of a Rhinoceros at Venice,* done circa 1751, which corresponds most closely to his description. It is in the National Gallery in London where Milosz might have seen it and remembered the animal differently.

p. 125. Phlegethon. A river of fire in Hades.

teraphim. Images or other objects representing primitive household gods.

p. 126. Gaupes. Fallen women.

p. 127. Hoffman. Liqueur d'Hoffman: a pharmaceutical concoction of equal quantities of ether and alcohol.

p. 129. Harpagon. The lead character in Molière's *L'Avare,* both avaricious and hypocritical.

p. 133. Philomel. Daughter of a king of Athens. Her brother-in-law had her tongue cut off, and she was later transformed into a nightingale.

p. 138. Nicolas Restif de la Bretonne [1734–1806]. A French writer who led an unconventional life and wrote scandalous books.

Louis Félicité de Brancas, comte de Lauraguais [1733–1824]. Renowned for his intelligence and his witticisms.

François de Colombières Briqueville [16th century]. Head of the French protestants at St-Lô, who refused to surrender.

p. 143. Paul Scarron (1610–1660). French poet, novelist, and playwright.

p. 151. Diafoirus. Father and son, both ignorant and pretentious physicians, characters in Molière's *Le Malade Imaginaire.*

Rowena. Celtic name meaning bright-haired; heroine in *Ivanhoe.*

p. 163. Restif [de la Bretonne]. Jean-Jacques [Rousseau].

p. 164. *Calli* and *campielli.* Venetian dialect for *streets* and *small squares.*

p. 170. Phoebe. Name for the moon, sometimes used instead of Artemis.

p. 171. l'abbé de Rancé. Trappist reformer [1626–1700], known for his rigorous morality.

p. 178. Manfredonia. A city in ancient Italy.

p. 179. Paraclete. Holy Spirit. Also, Monastery founded by Abèlard where Hèloïse was abbess.